SENSE AND SENSIBILITY IN HEALTH CARE

SENSE AND SENSIBILITY IN HEALTH CARE

Edited by
MARSHALL MARINKER
Visiting Professor of General Practice, UMDS, London and Advisor in Health Care Policy and Medical Education, MSD Ltd

BMJ
Publishing Group

First published in 1996
by the BMJ Publishing Group, BMA House,
Tavistock Square, London WC1H 9JR

British Library Cataloguing in Publication Data

A catalogue record for this book is available
from the British Library

ISBN 0-7279-1111-2

Typeset, printed and bound in Great Britain by
Latimer Trend and Company Ltd, Plymouth

Contents

Contributors

Richard Bradbury, Research Assistant, NHS Centre for Reviews and Dissemination, University of York

Graham Buckley, Director, Scottish Council for Postgraduate Medical and Dental Education, Edinburgh

Anna Coote, Deputy Director, Institute for Public Policy Research, London

June Crown, President, Faculty of Public Health Medicine

Vikki A Entwistle, Research Fellow, NHS Centre for Reviews and Dissemination, University of York

Louise Gunning-Schepers, Institute of Social Medicine, Academic Medical Centre, University of Amsterdam, The Netherlands

Lesley J Pehl, Research Fellow, NHS Centre for Reviews and Dissemination, University of York

John Spiers, Health Policy Adviser, The Social Market Foundation; Chairman, The Patients' Association; Visiting Fellow, King's Fund Management College, and NHS Staff College, Wales

Kieran Sweeney, General Practitioner, St Leonard's Medical Practice, Exeter, Devon

Ian S Watt, Dissemination Manager, NHS Centre for Reviews and Dissemination, University of York

Preface

The future health of the NHS, the achievement of the most accessible, efficient, effective, and humane health service possible, depends on open debate, and on the publication and scrutiny of a wide and original spectrum of informed opinions. In support of such open debate, and following the successful publication of a series of essays under the title *Controversies in Health Care Policies* (BMJ Publishing Group 1994), MSD* is delighted to have sponsored this further series of health policy papers.

As before, the aim has been to explore some controversial issues that often lie concealed behind the more headline grabbing political agendas. We invited Professor Marshall Marinker to identify a number of such topics, and to discuss these with relevant national organisations. In collaboration with six partner organisations, the issues were posed as questions, and think tanks were convened to broaden and deepen the discussion. The result is this collection of thought provoking and challenging essays.

In welcoming the publication I wish to express my warmest thanks to all those organisations and individuals involved, and very much hope that the appearance of *Sense and Sensibility in Health Care* will prove a stimulus to the further discussion and development of these ideas, and to the management of the paradoxes in policy making that its authors present.

Vincent Lawton,
Managing Director,
MSD UK Ltd

* Merck Sharp & Dohme is the UK subsidiary of Merck & Co. Inc., Whitehouse Station, New Jersey, USA.

1 Sense and sensibility

MARSHALL MARINKER

Introduction

This book contains six essays on aspects of health care policy that seemed, when they were first commissioned in 1995, to be of particular relevance to the rapidly changing health service in the United Kingdom. Five of them were commissioned under the aegis of national organisations concerned about the issues under review and were informed by think tank discussions. A sixth was in-dually commissioned.

The role of the participating national organisations was to identify the issues and endorse their relevance, to name the members of the think tanks, and to select the writer. All the authors invited comment on successive drafts of their work from a number of interested and informed individuals. Yet no single essay here represents a consensus view from any of the organisations involved, nor indeed from the members of the think tanks that were convened to take part in preliminary discussions.

My own involvement was to be the one common member of all the think tanks and, as required, to make brief editorial comments on some of the emerging drafts—but of a textual and not a conceptual nature. This afforded me an invaluable education in the ways in which some of the most intriguing questions about emerging health care policy are being discussed by informed leaders in the various health-related specialties. It also allowed me to see some camouflaged connections between the themes discussed. But the essays that follow do not, I believe, constitute a coherent whole. The achievement of such coherence was never part of the intention of this collection.

Rather these essays should be read as reports filed in some haste from the front lines, sometimes from behind the lines, of that no man's land where current concerned debate is going on. In this no man's land, the chairman of the BMA demands an annual increase of £6 billion of public funds for the service; both the major opposing political parties make the containment of public spending a key electoral promise; successive secretaries of state recite figures of increasing public expenditure and volume of activity (as though incanting a mantra for the public peace of mind), and the media publish stories of a cash strapped NHS allowing patients to die at the dictat of "accountants". From somewhere between the original assumptions and structures of the NHS and what is to come, these essays afford glimpses of the paradoxes and possibilities that are shaping not only the next few years but also the longer distant future.

The six essays that follow differ from one another in several significant ways. Although all of the think tanks were multidisciplinary in composition, chapters 2, 3, and 4 are written from the point of view of doctors. These deal not exclusively with the quality and outcomes of care but also with the nature of the medical task and with the status of professional roles, which are increasingly challenged and changing. Two of the essays constitute reflective commentaries from academic perspectives outside the NHS: chapter 5 is concerned with the way in which the most sensitive issues about choice and priorities are presented to the public; and chapter 6 looks at new ways in which the public's views can be explored and incorporated into health care planning at local level.

This chapter in particular contrasts starkly in style and tone with the deeply enigmatic chapter 7, by John Spiers. We are invited, like Alice, through the looking glass—though here it is the glass of the computer screen—into a very unfamiliar country. In fact this is the country of our immediate future, and the receipt of the chapter in draft confronted me with a particularly teasing editorial choice. The health service (and indeed the world) that is here described is in many ways bewilderingly different from anything that we have experienced hitherto. It is characterised not only by changed configurations (we have all become familiar with such iterative organisational changes in recent years) but by transformations in the nature of reality.

The style of the writing in this chapter is also disturbingly different from much of the literature on health policy with which the reader will be familiar. The arguments are not linear; the references are often oblique to the point the writer is making and are of unusual breadth. As editor I was, for example, delighted that the writer should assume without elucidation the reader's familiarity with Marcel Carné's 1945 cinema masterpiece *Les Enfants du Paradis*—a film that shaped my own sense of the intimate and the epic. This is not easy reading, and it is difficult at times not to lose one's bearings. But I have decided that to edit the original into some bland and solemn house style (the literary "political correctness" that most of us adopt in presenting our ideas in print) would be crucially to miss the point. The virtual hypertext language of this chapter, in its very unfamiliarity and contextual exuberance, conveys a powerful sense of the world that it describes.

Although I make no claim for coherence in the totality of the six topics chosen (still less in the picture that emerges), I detect the working out of two major contemporary themes. They present themselves, as I believe all health policy issues must, as paradoxes—the management of opposing goods: in the chapters concerned with public health advocacy, professionalism, and Evidence Based Medicine the paradox of sense and sensibility; in the chapters that deal with local democracy and the impact of information technology, the paradox of self and solidarity; in the chapter on the impact of the media, a bridging of both.

Sense and sensibility

Sensibility, as Jane Austen used the term in the title of her 1811 novel, referred to compassion for the suffering of others, to emotional sensitivity, and also to a certain refinement of taste. Sense, and hence the wit of her title, had a similar definition in its earlier English usage but subsequently referred to discerning the meaning of a word or text and later carried the additional burdens of "good" or "common" sense, thereby conveying the notion of sound judgment.

In her novels Jane Austen's young women are much concerned with making good marriages. These she represents as requiring a basis not only in affection and respect but also in financial security. Sensibility and sense are often at odds with one another, and indeed the tension between them drives the drama and sharpens the moral ambiguities. In the health service, as in the novels, these tensions and reconciliations test the private and public values of all the characters in the story. In the first four chapters that follow, these tensions are revealed in a number of different guises, but in their essence they reflect the same uncomfortable but necessary struggle to reconcile conflicting values.

Outside-in

A major task of the public health professional is to monitor the impact of government policy, industrial, commercial and other power and pressure groups, on the state of the public health. Perhaps the most powerful of these pressure groups, and one with some evident influence on health, is the NHS itself. But the past year has seen a fundamental structural change in the relationship of public health professionals and the authorities and boards and trusts which make up the service. This structural change has raised some quite profound anxieties about probity and loyalty.

The discipline of public health has been driven by two great engines: firstly, its scientific method—the engine of epidemiology that has been so powerful in revealing the causes of ill health; and, secondly, its crusading spirit—the deep concern for fairness and so advocacy for public health (the central theme of chapter 2).

Given the new corporate structure of the various components of the NHS introduced in 1990, how can the roles of public health director (that is, manager) be reconciled with that of advocate for the public health? The manager has corporate concerns and loyalties. The manager is an insider. The advocate must, in the very nature of things, be prepared to criticise, to oppose the system. For that purpose the manager must stand outside. The directors of public health, in their new guises as corporate players, feared that they were being turned outside in.

The NHS has been re-engineered in recent years to create something like a business relationship between the commissioners or purchasers (the authorities and fundholders) and the providers (trusts, general practices, and so on). Quality is expected to result, as it does in the commercial world, from contractual tensions and from the marketing edge between competing suppliers.

Crown and Gunning-Schepers are not concerned to debate the merits of this policy—perhaps because at the time of writing such changes as may be brought about by a change in government are thought unlikely to result in anything fundamentally different from the status quo. What they *are* concerned with is the way in which these recent arrangements may create conflicts of interest that go to the heart of the traditional mission of public health. For example, a director of public health in any of these organisations may in future find it hard to speak out critically in a way that will be at odds with the corporate codes of group confidentiality and loyalty and with what may now be considered the interests of the organisation as competitor.

The discussion and conclusion in this chapter provide an informative glimpse of a profession in transition, and this is particularly illuminating because, for the foreseeable future, rapid transition is likely to be the permanent condition of all the stakeholders in health care. This transition is not only a matter of the "natural" development of a discipline or a professional group. It may actually involve a realignment in tasks and roles such that the changes are no longer ones of degree or detail but of fundamental substance. In the light of other chapters in this collection concerned with professional futures the appearance of this subtext was informative.

For example, in the think tank discussions much was made of the need to keep in mind that most professionals in public health care were not in fact medical practitioners and that public health *medicine* should be recognised as a component of the broader discipline of public health. What then was the particular contribution of medicine to the pursuit of the public health?

The possibility exists, given the velocity of technical and social transformation, that some traditional professional groups will disappear. This is perhaps most likely to occur in groups that have become almost wholly dependent on a particular way of looking at morbidity (for example, psychiatry) or on the exploration of a particular technology (for example, radiology). The less dependent on particular technologies and the wider the role and remit (for example, in the cases of public health medicine and general practice) the more robust and adaptable the group. Of course professional groups can and do adapt, but if they fail then it is likely that something valuable and irreplaceable will be lost to practice.

In the case of public health medicine this "something" is neither the *sense* of epidemiology nor the *sensibility* of advocacy for fairness. Rather it is the way in which the two may be confidently held in productive tension. The authors identify the need (given the uncertainties of science and the vagaries of human behaviour) to "go beyond the evidence" and of the need to combine what they call "marketing as well as science". They describe *public health intuition* in the face of evidential uncertainty as an analogue of the personal physician's *clinical acumen.* The importance of this mysterious acumen in the carrying out of the clinical task much concerned the think tank members and authors of the two subsequent chapters (Graham Buckley and Kieran Sweeney). They are all talking about making sense of sense and sensibility.

Reality is made not given

Just as the public health advocates have had to adjust to being turned outside in, so increasingly the hospital clinicians look around their once familiar institutions and are unsure of their role and writ in its governance and their practice. In the past, hospitals and authorities were served by administrators. There was little doubt in the minds of most doctors that in the doctor–administrator relationship, if the administrator was the civil servant it was the doctor who was the minister of state or at least a member of the government.

Today the various components of the health service are managed not administered. Although the differences between management and administration may seem to be so subtle as to defy analysis, the difference is evidently *felt.* One consequence of the substitution of the word "administrator" with the word "manager" has been a sense that such managerial values as efficiency and competitiveness are now sharply discordant with such traditional professional ones as beneficence, advocacy, and effectiveness. Pellagrino is cited as describing equity and utility as "second order" imperatives for the physician. Although the managerial values are by no means necessarily at odds with the professional ones, there is new space for confusion and mischief.

The case of Jaymee Bowen illustrates this (and is dealt with extensively in chapter 5). This young girl suffered from a form of leukaemia that had failed to respond to a bone marrow transplant. In the clinical judgment of her doctors she would be greatly more harmed than helped by a second bone marrow transplant. Yet somehow this clinical judgment had to be underwritten by a higher managerial judgment concerning affordability and opportunity cost—with the consequent furore in the media.

The medical profession has long been fairly comfortable with three traditional obligations: to the patient, to the body politic of the profession, and to the public. Now, however, there is a new, or newly perceived, obligation which seems suddenly to have come into such sharp focus throughout the industrialised nations as they experiment with a variety of forms of prepaid managed care. This is the corporate obligation of the clinician to the institution. It can be seen to conflict with the fiduciary relationship to the patient, with the development of the interests of the profession as guild or discipline, and with the public interest. These conflicts may be compounded as new private sector stakeholders and players enter the NHS field.

The key to resolving this new conflict may not, of course, lie primarily in a reconsideration of the nature of professionalism. Of course professionalism may be redefined by a changing environment of care, but the resolution of conflicting obligations may lie less in rethinking professional values than in rethinking the organisations. I am not advocating yet another "reorganisation of the service" as a displacement therapy for governments trapped in the vice of rising cost-demand and relatively unyielding public budgets. Rather, I want to provoke a deeper consideration of how the organisations in which we work—that we have inherited and devised—delimit the reach of our capabilities and imaginations.

In his original monograph *Images of Organization* Gareth Morgan describes the pervasive power of metaphor on the way in which we think and behave and create.[1] Metaphor is intrinsic to our developed use of language. Medicine, for example, is much described in military terms: doctors *combat* the infections caused by *invading* bacteria with a powerful *armementarium* of antibiotics. In similar vein we use medical metaphors to refer to the national economy: we describe the currency as *ailing* and the stringent fiscal measures that follow as *strong medicine.* Critics of the medical profession tend to speak of *the medical mafia*, a metaphor that promises rich extrapolations.

Metaphor allows us to see one reality as though it were another, it disrupts expectation and experience with fresh perspectives, it springs the surprises that constitute the discoveries of science and the novelties of art. The exploration of metaphor forms a central tool in the contemporary analysis of art, linguistics, theoretical physics, psychoanalytical theory, social theory, and much else.

Morgan's contribution is to apply the method of metaphorical analysis to the theory of organisations.

He develops an interesting taxonomy, and it is no part of my purpose here to give anything other than the merest indication of his thesis. His typology, although heavily influenced by neo-Freudian theory, presents us with images of the organisations within which we work that seem part of common experience and (in a literal sense) *strangely* familiar. For example, his first image of organisation is the familiar one of the organisation as "machine", with its emphasis on central control, explicit rules, rigid discipline, uniformity, specialisation, and predictability. This is, he argues, still the dominant mode.

Another metaphor is the organisation as "organism", characterised by a concern to preserve its internal environment while at the same time discovering ecological niches by continuously interacting with and adapting to the changing external environment. Yet another describes the organisation as "brain"—each component acting as a microcosm and hologram of the whole; each separate part carrying within itself the entire repertoire of organisational structure and responses.

In all of this Morgan could be describing any of the NHS authorities and trusts and fundholders familiar to us. Moreover, he enables us to recognise them not in the sense that any one of them could be categorised as "machine" or "organism" or "brain", however tempted the reader may be to make such analyses. Rather, any of the organisations in which we work can be understood afresh in the light of any and all of these (and other) metaphors.

From the standpoint of much that is written in this collection, Morgan's most intriguing metaphor is what he terms the organisation as "psychic prison". Here the members and their endeavours are constantly trapped by archaic memories of the organisation's real or believed history. Drawing on Jungian imagery he quotes Mitroff as suggesting that organisational life can be understood in terms of the relationship between fools, magicians, warriors, high priests, lovers, and other symbolic characters.[2] It is perhaps no accident that the think tank of public health professionals, contemplating their positions as newly corporate members of authorities and trusts, describes one of the roles as "poet in residence".

If the idea of medical professionalism is to survive and develop in the corporate NHS, doctors must of course adapt, but they can also adapt their organisations, not least by forming adventurous alliances. This can happen only if they are prepared to reinvent their organisations in the light of more appropriate metaphors—my own would include the hospital as production of grand opera and primary care as, perhaps, street theatre. The process by which this is brought about, Morgan describes intriguingly as "imaginization". He reminds us that no matter how long and powerful the tradition of the status quo, "reality is made not given".

The problem with evidence

Nowhere was the paradox of sense and sensibility more painfully experienced than in the group of GPs considering the impact of Evidence Based Medicine (EBM). So far, although much has been written about the organisational growth of general practice in the United Kingdom, its patterns of recorded morbidities and work load, there has been no analytical account of the way in which the GP has developed a unique vision of "the diagnosis". We still require a retrospective that charts the experiences of NHS GPs, the idiosyncratic characteristics of practice—the openness and relative informality of access (by the patient to the doctor's surgery and by the doctor to the patient's home); the contrast between the average brevity of individual encounters and longevity of doctor–patient relationships; the parsimonious use of laboratory and imaging investigation, and so on—have shaped the doctor's understanding of "what is wrong". Some of these variables were already established in prewar private and panel general practice and have changed little during the 50 year history of the NHS. But from the start of the service they marked out the landscape, they determined the doctor's field of clinical vision, they gave a language to describe if not yet to explain.

The changing focus in that field of vision was determined, however, by other factors extraneous to practice. For most of the past 50 years, general practice as a clinical craft has been driven by a series of fresh insights, views of the clinical situation from such various disciplines as epidemiology, demography, sociology, psychoanalysis, and social psychology. The influence of the social and behavioural sciences on what Foucault calls the doctor's "gaze" was exerted for the most part by a small number of talented, articulate, and charismatic figures.[3] But the social and behavioural sciences were not long permitted their preferred pastime of theoretical social comment and critique.

The motivation to reconsider what had been traditionally taught in the medical school came entirely from the GPs themselves. The new insights did not long remain the separate province of the social sciences. They were incorporated into the medical gaze itself. In the words of one of the key objectives of vocational training endorsed by the Royal College of General Practitioners *all* of the doctor's diagnoses were to be composed "*simultaneously* in physical, psychological and social terms" (my italics).[4] The core of the discipline of general practice was formed by this total fusion of clinical sense and sensibility.

Many saw in this a paradigm shift in medical theory, almost certainly too ambitious a claim. But it was a defining transformation, and it created both a solution and a problem. It encouraged a truly holistic practice to develop, such that the disease and the person could not easily be dissected in the name of a spurious biological objectivity. The doctor, the patient, and the illness were ineluctably linked, composed together as the mingled object of the medical gaze in general practice. The problem, which is now becoming more clearly apparent, is that general practice has only half completed the paradigm shift that some of its academics and polemicists have proclaimed.

What still remain largely outside the frame of reference are the diseases themselves, their names and classifications. We still await a means of study beyond epidemiology to map a no man's land of conditions, anywhere between the earliest appearance of symptoms and diagnostic closure. These diseases can only be spoken of, or must remain outside the clinical discourse, according to the syntactic rules and vocabulary of a language which was developed first in the postmortem room and subsequently in the laboratory; a language that cannot express what the GPs and their patients require to be articulated.

Evidence Based Medicine (EBM) is a relatively recent term coined to identify a method and system of presenting to the practising clinician the best evidence on clinical effectiveness from research reports which have been expertly scrutinised to ensure the quality of the methods used.[5] The system is more fully described and discussed in chapter 4, and here the reader may quickly detect in Sweeney's appraisal and critique of EBM, a reservation amounting almost to suppressed hostility. Throughout the discussions, these negative feelings ran high in many of the members of the think tank, most of whom came from general practice. Why?

I do not intend in this introductory essay to review the arguments put forward in the chapter. Many of them have been refuted by some of the leading protagonists of Evidence Based Medicine (themselves from general practice) in private correspondence with me. They claim that, in what is presented here, the methods and system have been misrepresented or misunderstood. Rather, my concern here is to ask why so many leading GPs react in this strongly ambivalent way to what must surely be regarded as a substantial contribution to the enhancement of clinical standards. What is going on?

There are, I believe, a number of sources of this anger and anxiety. The most important lies in the perception that the language of Evidence Based Medicine somehow misses the point of the clinical encounter in primary general clinical practice. There is added fear that what begins as "best information" on which to base a decision can easily be transformed into contractual instruments designed to control not simply facilitate the management of the patient. There is a suspicion that clinical judgment will be supplanted with protocols and algorithms of diagnosis and treatment that will constitute (perhaps legally) the acceptable and mandated medical response to illness. These may well be quite unrealistic fears (the progenitors and proponents of EBM would certainly deny such dirigiste ambitions), but they are quite widely felt and expressed.

Another cause of disquiet in general practice about EBM lies in its implications for the future role of GPs. As specialisms become truly successful in the development of innovations they reach a point at which previously difficult diagnoses and treatments no longer require specialist intervention. That is to say, that they become routines. Paul Beeson writing in the *Annals of Internal Medicine* observed ". . . practice specialties thrive in situations where something can be offered, but where that something is complex, and only partially effective".[6] This contrasts with his statement "I am impressed by the evidence that the introduction of simple curative treatments means trouble for a practice specialty". Just so.

Much that was recently in the sole clinical province of specialists has become part of routine general practice. But the dissemination of technical competence, particularly in the new age of information technology, can no longer be confined by the interests of a particular craft or guild. Standards and protocols in the management of the major diseases, consequent on the information being generated by EBM, may make possible and desirable a quite radical new skill mix in primary medical care. This is one of the themes explored in chapter 7.

In trying to make sense out of the evidence about diagnosis and treatment in general practice, the protagonists of EBM have highlighted what still eludes the researchers and are stirring up the deepest sensibilities.

Jaymee's story

The media presentation and discussion of the way in which the NHS responded to Jaymee Bowen, set out in chapter 5, reveal a deep wish (perhaps on the part of most of us) for a simple and compassionate view of health care policy—one that opposes virtue and vice, fairness and injustice, hope and despair, life and death. The story of Jaymee Bowen is the very stuff of the romantic and heroic novel. In many ways it was not hard to see in Jaymee something of many of Austen's heroines: feisty, irrepressible, angry, reflective, and ironic. Jaymee was a very private self but at the same time a public icon, a heroine, a victim, a cause, and a field of discourse.

The Jaymee Bowen story crystallised a general public unease that the founding principles of the NHS might no longer be intact. Furthermore, there was a distinct anxiety that somehow there was a failure of truth telling on which any confidence in a professional relationship and a public service must rest. There was a growing sense, in the light of this and other stories, that we had all better take some compass bearings by which to determine the future direction of health policy. Yet, what if the principles and values of a public service (or for that matter of a professional relationship) are not universal? What if they are, rather, quite contingent on context, time, and place?

In fact the NHS was introduced into a very different United Kingdom from the one that it serves today: it catered for a different public and a different patient. In the years immediately after the war bread and other food staples were still rationed. The accepted hallmark of austere good taste was a design of furniture labelled "Utility". The car industry still offered the 1930s Henry Ford choice of black paint work or black, and there were long waiting lists for delivery. Queues were part of a social choreography that expressed a public ethic of fair shares in response to scarcity. In a world in which rationing was agreed to be the only rational response to limited goods, health care rationing could not be distinguished from the ambient culture. The social scientists had scarcely begun to mount their devastating critique of professional paternalism. Benign paternalism was the unquestioned central tenet of the design and delivery of the 1948 health service.

The contrast with the ambient culture of the 1990s need hardly be emphasised. In contemporary Britain, citizenship is confused with consumerism and democracy with marketing. Choice and individualism are elevated to the status of moral imperatives. At the time of purchase, such is the range of optional extras offered on even the most popular mass production models that each new car is perceived to be (and may well be) *uniquely* customised. The consumer is characterised not only by the right to choice but also by entitlement to redress. At the time of writing this, a patient who was told by his doctors that he had only three months to live but has survived for over two years under their care is attempting to sue them for the anxiety and stress caused by their prognosis and his unanticipated life.

We hear much party political debate in the 1990s about the advantages and dangers of privatising public services. What too often escapes our notice is that in developed economies, like that of the United Kingdom, there has been an inexorable privatisation of public morality. And the media discussion of Jaymee Bowen reflects this.

The key moral question, in terms of the use of limited resources, was posed here by the availability of a relatively expensive treatment that offered extremely unlikely benefit to an individual patient. This extremely unlikely benefit, however, could scarcely have been more substantial—the potential saving of a child's life. A public discussion of how to think about the opportunity cost in all this, however, is unthinkable without an assumption of social solidarity. And a preference for the language of health economics over that of clinical appropriateness reflects a scale of values that holds health care to be a commodity: a noun not a verb.

A public prepared to invest tens of millions of pounds each week on the odds offered by the National Lottery may well have a view of the probabilities and risks involved in the so called experimental treatments mooted in response to Jaymee's leukaemia quite different from that of clinical researchers and health economists. A single lottery ticket is no wager—it is the purchase of a dream. Was this the purchase (the "experimental" treatment) that the tabloids and others were urging—the dream of Jaymee's cure? If so it reflected a common human preference for sensibility over sense. It also represented the eclipse of solidarity in the shadow of self.

So strong was the instinct to "save" Jaymee by going to the outer margins of possibility that little regard was given by the media to the suffering that lay beyond the margins. And as life itself becomes ever more medicalised it seems no longer acceptable or sufficient simply to grant God His usual exoneration from blame for suffering and death. Yet death, which can hardly be spoken of in the same breath as medicine, must be somebody's fault. Someone has to shoulder the blame. In what the tabloids made a gladiatorial contest and a compellingly serialised novel, fair sensibility (the compassion felt by the reader and viewer for Jaymee and her father) was defeated by cruel sense (the evidence from the sciences of medicine and health economics). And to complicate matters there was an important subplot to the story of sense and sensibility: the story of the paradox of self and solidarity. This subplot becomes more evident still in the next two chapters.

Vox populi

It is not only in the news or documentary programmes that television (arguably our most potent communication medium at the present time) deals with the NHS and its policies and management. Current TV drama series like *Casualty*, *Cardiac Arrest*, and *Peak Practice* take up the same dramatic themes of choice and consequence. Their analogues in the United States like *ER* also convey the messages that the dilemmas may be not only a product of a particular government or its political complexion in respect of public or private funding but also of something in the very grain of human illness, modern medicine, and the institutionalisation of care. Or at least that the contingencies are not as parochial as might be imagined. How the public can better reflect on all this and on their personal experiences of health care, how they can directly influence the shape and quality of the service, is the subject of chapter 6.

What Coote identifies is a democratic deficit in the NHS, such that local communities have insufficient influence on the nature and qualities of local provision and no sense that those who provide the service are demonstrably accountable to them. What is said to be missing is a sense of local "ownership".

Several possible mechanisms for achieving this are described and discussed. Of course, greater local democracy creates its own dilemmas. It opens up the possibility of widening local variations of provision and practices within the state system and even the possibility of raising local taxes to pay for special local health care needs or desires. This can, of course, compromise such principles as equity and fairness at the national level, but it also intriguingly begs the question of the size and boundaries of the playing field that is to be kept level.

On the other hand an NHS based on local government might well encourage the building of innovative engines, such that experiments in the delivery of health care can be tailored to the peculiar character and culture of local communities. As I write this, one major provincial city, Newcastle-upon-Tyne, is acting on my suggestion that they apply for the status of a NHS Social Enterprise Zone. A group of partners composed of the city council, the health authority, hospital and community trusts, businesses, trades union, and sporting interests and others is drawing up a multi-agency proposal for radical and cooperative experimentation in health care.

As a prerequisite they are asking for the suspension of constraining national regulations and guidelines to allow a truly local approach. The city will provide a social laboratory for NHS development, and the experiments will be evaluated by the appropriate local university departments.

Local communities in the post-industrial society are set to become increasingly heterogeneous.[7] But there is a further paradox here. These communities are unlikely to become internally homogenous in terms of their health care priorities. They will continue to be composed of a complex collection of competing minorities, identified by age, sex, disease, disability, vulnerability, and so on. Democracy serves the interest of majorities well, but is less sensitive to those of minorities. Nor are hard choices about priorities, innovations, exclusions, and so on best left to the vagaries of the political cockpit.

None the less, the resolution of the paradox of politics and professionalism may better be achieved at local than at national level, and (as Coote describes) by more sensitive methods than the ballot box. A locally created and accountable service, delimited only by a national framework of public funding and ethical imperatives, may serve us better, if for no other reason than that the errors committed will not be massive and nationally uniform and by the nature of their diversity will offer us the chance of learning more rapidly from them.

Anna Coote's chapter is concerned with new and better ways of making the voice of the local population heard in the monitoring of the service and in the generation of policy. John Spiers, in his essay on where the promise of information technology will take us, is not concerned with the empowerment of communities by local democratic means but with the empowerment of individuals by means of global informatics.

Self and solidarity

There could scarcely have been a more stark contrast in assumptions about the nature of self, society, personal freedom, and mutual obligation than those found in these last two chapters. The very languages they use are foreign to one another, they belong to different countries. The problem for the reader is that if we do not simultaneously inhabit both of them now, we very soon shall.

In the introductory chapter to a previous collection of essays on health policy I quoted Richard Rorty's postmodernist monograph *Contingency, Irony and Solidarity.*[8] I was concerned then to embrace the idea of the "contingency" of our language (principles, values, assumptions) in talking about medicine and science and health, in any one particular place and time. Also, I urged Rorty's sense of the virtues of "irony", the willingness to respect the language of others, and (more difficult) to accept that it is impossible to mount an adequate critique of the ideas expressed in a contingent language by using that same language. More directly, it is not sufficient to examine critically the assumptions of, say, general practice in the United Kingdom, in what I earlier described as its own distinctive and defining language.

The chance contiguity here of the chapters by Coote and Spiers, allows me to return to Rorty's monograph in search of the possibilities for mutual caring and social obligation in this postmodern world. I should, however, preface this by admitting that the arrival of this world is by no means universally recognised, and even where it is, by no means universally welcomed. Charlton described "... the anomalous position of medicine in contemporary culture—an island of rationalistic modernity floating in a shifting sea of subjective postmodernity—a castle of objectivity besieged by the forces of relativistic cynicism."[9] What is, in fact, anomalous about medicine is that it is at once both island and sea.

In the concluding chapter of his monograph, Rorty confronts the possibility of a social solidarity that does not rely on such religious or philosophical precepts as moral duty or common humanity but is consistent with a contingent view of morality and is the more robust for being so grounded. He opens his argument by observing, "If you were a Jew in the period when the trains were running to Auschwitz, your chances of being hidden by your gentile neighbours were greater if you lived in Denmark or Italy than if you lived in Belgium", and he asks why. His conclusion is not that one national group has a greater moral sensitivity than another but that for "contingent" (that is, historical) reasons the Danes or the Italians were at that time more likely than the Belgians to see their neighbour not as a Jew but as "someone like me"—a fellow Milanese or Jutlander or member of the same profession or union. Rorty suggests that social solidarity comes from a recognition that the dissimilarities between people and groups are insignificant compared with the similarities. Solidarity is an extension of the idea of the self.

Spiers' view of the future does not refer to the sense of social solidarity given voice by local democracy that informs Coote's essay. But it does hold open an alternative road to solidarity and moral progress in health care. It envisages a web of individual selves on the Internet, linked by common experiences and expressions of suffering and care, each of whom can become "someone like me".

The collection of essays that follows is offered in the hope of shedding some light on the journey to a future NHS, which manages the paradox of sense and sensibility in health care practice and the paradox of self and solidarity in a service which is at once appropriate, effective, and just.

1 Morgan G. *Images of organisation.* Beverly Hills: Sage, 1986.
2 Mitroff I. *Stakeholders of the mind.* San Francisco: Jossey-Bass, 1984.

3 Foucault M. *Birth of the clinic.* London: Tavistock, 1973.
4 The Royal College of General Practitioners. *The future general practitioner.* London: RCGP, 1973.
5 Davidoff F, Haynes B, Sackett D, *et al.* Evidence based medicine. *BMJ* 1995; **310**:1085–6.
6 Beeson PB. The natural history of medical sub-specialties. *Ann Intern Med* 1980; **93**:624–6.
7 Toffler A. *Future shock.* London: Bodley Head, 1970.
8 Rorty R. *Contingency irony and solidarity.* Cambridge: Cambridge University Press, 1989.
9 Charlton B. Medicine and post-modernity. *J R Soc Med* 1993;**86**:497–9.

The Partner:

The Faculty of Public Health Medicine, Royal College of Physicians, London

The Question:

How can the role of public health advocate be reconciled with that of NHS corporate player?

The Writers:

Dr June Crown, President, Faculty of Public Health Medicine
Professor L Gunning Schepers, Institute of Social Medicine, University of Amsterdam

Think Tank Members:

Dr Sheila Adam, Head of Mental Health and NHS Community Care, Department of Health
Professor John Ashton, Regional Director of Public Health, NHS Executive (North West)
Dr Ian Baker, Consultant in Public Health Medicine, Avon Health Authority
Professor John Butler, Head of Department of Social and Public Policy and Social Work, University of Kent
Dr Jacqueline Chambers, Director of Public Health, North Birmingham Health Authority
Dr Michael Gill, Director of Public Health, Brent & Harrow Health Authority
Dr Sian Griffiths, Director of Public Health, Oxfordshire Health Authority, and Treasurer, Faculty of Public Health Medicine
Dr Deirdre Hine (Chair), Chief Medical Officer, Welsh Office
Professor Marshall Marinker, Visiting Professor of General Practice, UMDS, London and Advisor in Health Care Policy and Medical Education, MSD Ltd
Professor James McEwan, Professor of Public Health, University of Glasgow, and Academic Registrar, Faculty of Public Health Medicine
Dr David Stuart, Director of Public Health, Eastern Health and Social Services Board
Ms Beth Wagstaff, Deputy Chief Executive, Hertfordshire County Council

2 The challenge to public health advocacy

JUNE CROWN, LOUISE GUNNING-SCHEPERS

Public health—The science and art of preventing disease, prolonging life, and promoting health through the organised efforts of society

Public health practitioner—A person, from any discipline or professional group, including medicine, whose job is primarily concerned with improving public health

Public health medicine—That branch of medicine which specialises in public health

Public health physician—A doctor trained in public health medicine
Director of public health—A public health physician who is the chief medical adviser to a health authority in the NHS and an executive member of the authority

Introduction

The practice of public health has always involved tensions and potential conflict. On the one hand, there is a professional obligation to argue for changes which improve health. On the other hand, the public health practitioner usually works at a senior level within an organisation with wider and sometimes conflicting responsibilities. As public health improvements are achieved by the "organised efforts of society", the corporate role can add not just credibility but also feasibility to the advocacy role.

A recent example in the United Kingdom is the campaign to reduce waiting lists for hospital treatment. Considerable financial and human resources have been allocated to the achievement of waiting list targets in the NHS. Although this is a desirable aim, many public health professionals consider that greater health gain would have been produced if these resources had been invested in other ways. They have, nevertheless, assisted with the work on waiting lists as part of their contribution to the corporate agenda.

The recent restructuring of the NHS in the United Kingdom has drawn attention to the role of public health in a changing policy context and particularly the potential conflict between public health advocacy and organisational corporacy. Regional health authorities in England have become regional offices of the NHS Executive and regional directors of public health have become civil servants. At the district level, directors of public health are executive members of the health authorities in which the managerial imperatives often do not coincide with public health priorities; the numbers of public health staff are limited by management cost controls; and the major task at present is contracting for health services. Can the different roles that public health professionals have traditionally taken be easily reconciled in this new corporate environment or should we anticipate increasing tensions between these different roles?

The potential problems were highlighted in discussions with regional directors of public health as they contemplated incorporation into the civil service and in the medical press in late 1995. The issue, however, is not new. It has been of concern and dealt with in different ways since public health was established as an independent specialty. The foundations of public health in the United Kingdom were laid in the 1840s with the appointment of the first medical officers of health by local authorities. Their tasks then were to tackle the health problems arising from rapid urbanisation—such as inadequate sanitation and housing—cynically described as "protecting the rich from the diseases of the poor". At the outset, they were paid high salaries and were prohibited from undertaking private medical practice so as to avoid conflict of interest. Until 1974, when medical officers were brought into the NHS as area medical officers or district community physicians, they were protected from dismissal by their employing authorities to ensure that they were free to give professional advice in the public interest even when it was unwelcome to town councils. Many annual reports from medical officers were outspoken on issues of education, employment, and town planning as well as on health care matters such as local hospital provision and communicable disease control.

In the United Kingdom public health medicine is currently statutorily represented at national and local levels. The chief medical officers for England, Scotland, Wales, and Northern Ireland are civil servants who advise government across all departments on matters which affect the health of the population. At the local level, each district has a director of public health, who is an executive member of the authority and its chief medical adviser. The new districts in England and Wales which now, like those in Scotland and Northern Ireland, combine the responsibilities of the former health authorities with those of the family health services authorities have been described as "public health organisations". Their task is to assess the health of the population and to monitor and improve health within an agreed budget.

The development of an NHS led by primary care and the extension of GP fundholding seems to provide an opportunity to realise the public health potential of the new district health authority. But at the same time there are concerns that the changes may reduce the scope to achieve the necessary reallocation of resources. If fundholding really puts the responsibility for purchasing services in accordance to the population's needs with the GPs, the position of the director of public health in the new NHS system will certainly be different. The new context may encourage and enable a return to some of the more traditional public health functions.

Several current developments and initiatives illustrate the possible areas in which public health practitioners in the future may become involved. All of them derive from the professional obligation to protect the health of the population, particularly the most vulnerable groups.

There are several current issues where the health practitioner might be expected to assess the public health implications and to set them out clearly and firmly.

The interest of pharmaceutical companies in developing programmes of managed care for certain diseases gives rise to concern about issues such as equity of access, appropriateness of care, and choice. The increased role of the private sector in the provision of care in nursing homes raises questions about the services provided for vulnerable people by staff who are not always required to participate in audit and continuing education programmes to maintain their professional skills and standards. The Private Finance Initiative is expected to improve the quality of capital developments in the public sector and to speed up their completion. It is linked with the privatisation of some non-clinical services, such as cleaning and catering, however, which none the less have considerable effects on the quality of care, with potentially serious impacts on control of infection and nutrition.

In this chapter we explore some of the functions that public health professionals have traditionally undertaken in the health system in the United Kingdom and examine the possible developments and tensions which may arise in the changing circumstances of the NHS. The tensions may never be resolved. We therefore deal with some of the principles which should inform the establishment of safeguards that will be necessary, whatever the organisational setting, if the comprehensive role of public health, including advocacy is to be sustained and developed.

Although we are focusing on the United Kingdom, it is important to recognise that these tensions are not unique to the United Kingdom. In the context of reforms of health systems, similar discussions are taking place across Europe and in many other developed countries.

The functions of the public health practitioner

The specialty of public health includes many disciplines—such as medicine, economics, education, and engineering—all of which can contribute to improvements in health. Recruits to the discipline come with a range of motivations—predominantly scientific, political, managerial—linked with a commitment to health. All would probably subscribe to the key medical ethical principles of autonomy, beneficence, non-maleficence, and justice. The forces which bind public health practitioners are, however, not only their professional skills. They include the commom values of equity, social justice, and the value and dignity of all communities. These values are often manifest in a commitment to change and in advocacy for the underserved and disadvantaged groups in society.

It is these often strongly felt common values, this self imposed role as the conscience of the health system, the advocate of the public, that can lead to conflict when the public health professional has to function within a corporate structure where other interests may have to take priority. Although we will concentrate on the constraints felt by many public health professionals who work within the NHS, it must be acknowledged that there are other organisations in which similar problems may be experienced. Academics have to deal with the difficult issues which arise when a university is offered substantial funds for much needed posts or research programmes from donors who are considered to be inappropriate because their business activities are harmful to health. A current example is the debate on the establishment of a chair funded by a tobacco manufacturer. Pharmaceutical funding can raise similar concerns. Similarly, public health practitioners seek to support the corporacy of the medical profession through the Faculty of Public Health Medicine's membership of the Academy of Medical Royal Colleges, while maintaining their primary concern for the health of the population rather than the diseases of individual patients.

It has been suggested that clinicians deal with problems which are largely unchanging by using new techniques, while public health physicians tackle new tasks and problems with techniques which are essentially unchanged. Put another way, the creativity of clinicians is channelled into new approaches to existing problems which have to be introduced and tested with extreme caution; the creativity of public health physicians lies in the early identification of new problems, the innovative analysis of their causal determinants, and the ability to bring about change within complex organisations. The instruments of change—assessing the evidence, convincing others, mediating between opposing interests, and occasionally using regulation—remain constant even though the focus of required change will differ. The primary objective remains to prevent disease, prolong life, and promote health through the organised efforts of society. In that process the public health practitioner has many parts to play: to define what needs to change; to identify a method by which change can be achieved and the people with the power to bring about change; to have the powers of persuasion to influence those people in favour of health.

Public health advocate

The public health practitioner has always been an advocate of the population's health, trying to introduce a public health perspective in the decision making at different levels. Traditionally the annual report of the director of public health is important in this respect as the opportunity for independent public statements on health. Great importance is attached to the maintenance of these reports, free of external editorial interference, as powerful agents of change as well as contributions to public archives. There is also the potential for disagreement in day to day activities such as board and executive meetings. A health authority or trust or indeed the NHS itself can under some circumstances feel threatened by the independent views of one of its public health professionals. This insider–outsider role of the public health professional is not only ambiguous but complex: authorities and trusts themselves may perceive the need for a public health advocate who observes, criticises, and monitors, while still remaining a part of the organisation.

This complex and ambiguous role can be identified at government level, where the power and resources of the tobacco, alcohol, and food industries—and their influence on ministers—have to be balanced by civil servants using evidence derived from research on such issues as cigarette advertising, levels of duty on alcohol and advice on "safe limits", and nutritional and animal husbandry practices. At local level, directors of public health may have to challenge influential local industries in relation to environmental damage; local authorities in relation to transport policy; or even the local NHS trust in relation to the promotion of the health of its employees.

The public health practitioner is not just the professional leader and advocate of programmes of health improvement but often also takes on the role of the voice of the public, the representative of those who use the services, and the champion of those with particular needs. The position he or she takes in a debate can be based on the professional assessment of consumers' best interests or understanding of public preferences arising from empowerment of users of the service and encouragement of consumers to influence their own health and health care.

In that case, however, advocacy implies values as well as science. It would be arrogant to assume that the values of public health practitioners take precedence over all others and that they are the sole guardians of public opinion. It has traditionally been the role of the public health professional, however, to consider the best interest of the total population even if that were to conflict with the interests of individual patients or to interfere with individual clinicians or managers. The role of guardian of the public interest has led some public health doctors to take on the role of the community representative. It remains difficult, however, to identify the most legitimate stakeholders on a particular issue and even harder to elicit the majority opinion rather than that of the activist.

The advocacy role must be an essential component of any organisation which seeks to improve health. The central public health concern for equity should be expressed through reports on inequalities in health and support for measures to reduce them. Public health advocates are expected to support the continuing battle againt smoking, establishing their own organisations as exemplars and promoting changes in policy at national and local levels. They should also keep on the agenda the problems of underprivileged and underserved groups, such as older people, ethnic minorities, and refugees. Public health advocates must also remain conscious of the breadth of health determinants and speak out on the implications of environmental, food, transport, fiscal, and other public policies.

Public health scientist

It is clear that the public health practitioner needs to have skill in measuring the health of the population, identifying possible health threats and evaluating measures aimed to improve health. It is for this reason that there has always been a great emphasis on the scientific basis for public health practice, the need for a close working relationship with academic public health, and sound training. Part of public health legitimacy comes from the sapiential authority of public health professionals. The analysis of health problems and the proposals for interventions should be based on scientific evidence. Public health practitioners have leading roles in the establishment of "evidence based practice" and the assessment of the effectiveness of clinical care.

The scientific role of public health practitioners is also essential to epidemiological investigations—for example, in the control of outbreaks of communicable disease, the investigation of disease clusters, such as leukaemia, and the analysis of health screening programmes.

Public health practice involves marketing as well as science, however, and sometimes needs to go beyond the evidence. There is a place for "intuition"—the public health equivalent of "clinical acumen", based on experience, and there is certainly no case for delaying action in situations where the hazards are negligible and possible benefits significant while waiting for the evidence to accumulate. For example, it would generally be considered sensible to reduce air pollution even though the relationship with respiratory disease may not yet be completely elucidated.

Public health manager

The public health practitioner also contributes as a manager with direct responsibility for promoting the population's health. This managerial role is a predominant one for the director of public health, who should take a leading role in shaping the strategy of the health authority. This responsiblity is also discharged through contributions to the corporate debate on priorities and resource allocation and through the provision of information to the organisation on health status and risks. More specifically, public health practitioners often have direct responsibility for some services, such as communicable disease control and screening services.

Public health networker

To achieve these direct health objectives public health practitioners must be able to bring together different interest groups. It is their ability to network at organisational, professional, and community levels that determines their success. The facilitative role is widely recognised as important but may be considered a personal skill rather than a professional achievement and is not the monopoly of public health practitioners. The ability to form alliances is, however, an essential element in implementation of public policy. Effective intersectoral action requires the skills now which differ from those which were appropriate in the past. There is no longer the automatic approval and acceptance of a doctor's professional status nor of the idea that health issues might overrule other interests. This is further reinforced by the epidemiological transition from infectious to chronic diseases. After all it is much easier to see why a public health doctor would need to be involved in analysing and combating an outbreak of tuberculosis than in changing food prices to achieve a change in diet conducive to preventing cardiovascular disease.

Corporate player

The concepts of corporacy in the NHS, and with it the function of the public health practitioner as corporate player continue to change. Before the introduction of the internal market the corporate body with which departments of public health identified included hospitals and community services. The director of public health worked closely with clinical colleagues on service developments, participated in audit, advised on medical staffing, and was a full member of medical committees. In some cases, the close involvement with the provision of health care was seen as a barrier to adequate public health activity because it was so time consuming. Elsewhere, it provided the opportunity for reorientation of health services towards health promotion and disease prevention.

Immediately after the reforms, the sometimes combative language of "the market" and the adversarial nature of some contract negotiations diminished the sense of identity that public health practitioners had with providers. The corporate body was the health authority, the purchaser, and the task was the assessment of needs and commissioning of services for a population of 200 000–300 000 people. This was often a "natural" community and the public health practitioner could aim for a corporate role as the surrogate for the consumer of services, the custodian of clinical standards, and the advocate of value rather than price in purchasing decisions and contracts—though the reality of the role was often different.

More recently in England and Wales, districts have merged, attaining populations of 500 000–700 000, with a broader geographical spread and less sense of natural community. Health authorities are now merging with family health services authorities and the NHS is to become a service led by primary care. The future role of health authorities is defined as "strategy, advice and monitoring". As more services are purchased by GP fundholders, the public health practitioner's corporate role will change again to reflect the new balance. In this new situation the responsibility for purchasing will be much more fragmented and the public health perspective may no longer be that of one geographically defined population but instead encompass a diversity of patient and population perspectives. A director of public health will increasingly have to shift emphasis from working with clinicians in hospitals and community services to working with general practitioners and other primary care professionals.

As "corporate" players public health practitioners will play their part in helping the authority to respond to central initiatives such as waiting lists, emergency admissions, and management cost controls. They will influence and then be expected to stand by the collective decisions on matters such as purchasing choices or the closure of clinical services.

Public health as the conscience of the organisation

As this sense of partnership with the executives of the NHS and involvement in the corporate structure grows it may be increasingly difficult for public health practitioners to fulfil the function of the "conscience of the organisation", "poet in residence", or the critic of the system. In this role, the public health practitioner holds up a mirror to the organisation itself and helps it to be self reflective about its aims and objectives, structures and processes.

The annual public health report is an important part of this function. It should include an honest assessment of progress towards targets that were set in previous years. It gives the opportunity to analyse successes and failures. It provides a platform for proposals aimed at improving health in a specific population, which will indicate the public health priorities for allocation of resources.

Activities of this kind are important for an organisation but not necessarily popular if they imply criticism from one who is expected to be a corporate player.

Tensions between the varied functions of public health practice

Over the years all these different public health functions have been taken on by public health practitioners. Some have concentrated on a scientific career in an academic setting, others have worked entirely in service departments. Increasingly professionals other than doctors have become important in public health practice. For example, interest in environmental threats has increased, more attention has been given to health education, and the health economists have taken a greater role in policy analysis. Their contribution has greatly increased the strength of the public health voice in public policy and in health policy.

It must also be recognised that public health advocacy is not the sole prerogative of public health professionals. Although the public and the media often still look for the authority of a doctor when seeking an opinion, many outstanding health advocates are found among clinicians, environmental health officers, voluntary organisations, trading standards officers, and social scientists. In many instances their legitimacy is at least as great, if not greater, than that of public health practitioners.

Within the NHS, however, the public health doctor has had to continue to combine all the different functions described above. As the context in which they have to work changes, the balance between the need for the different functions changes as well, sometimes creating new tensions. There has always been a very strong position for the director of public health because of their traditional role as the public health advocate, exemplified by the annual report. This opportunity to report independently on the population's health has been envied in many other countries where the public health voice is not as easily heard. As the pressures on health services resources become more evident and the unmet demands for care more apparent, however, there is a tendency to concentrate more on the allocation of resources within the health system and less on the wider intersectoral aspects of health promotion. Under the circumstances, the functions of advocate and corporate player may not go well together. The director may be constrained in criticising ill chosen priorities or marginalised for taking a strong advocacy role in the corporate setting. In addition, the perceived identification with NHS management may prejudice relationships with other clinicians.

Traditionally, public health physicians have been seen as intermediaries between clinicians and managers because of their combination of medical education and training in management. Their knowledge of epidemiology and statistics underpins their scientific analysis of health problems. In some instances, there may be difficulties with clinicians who consider that public health doctors have turned their back on patient care in favour of anonymous populations. At the same time a public health doctor possesses skills that are of interest to other physicians. This may entail professional skills such as knowledge of epidemiology and the managerial ability to make things happen. As the formal role of the district changes, as it becomes a public health organisation, and at the same time clinicians become more interested in evaluating interventions and better trained in epidemiology, the traditionally unique knowledge and skills of public health no longer seem to be limited to public health professionals.

The legitimacy of clinicians in relation to individual patient care is easily established. In most instances the patient consults the clinician voluntarily and consents to treatment. The clinician is expected to offer what is best for the patient and to be an advocate for improvements in his or her particular service in the interests of the patients. The legitimacy of the public health practitioner is harder to define. In some instances, there is a demand for public health intervention—for example, in the control of communicable disease. More often, however, the public feel pressured or even oppressed by public health exhortations to stop smoking, drink less, abandon the car, and avoid "fast foods". Public health practitioners may be seen as taking a moral high ground, which, despite protestations, takes little account of public opinion.

Historically the civil service was established to serve the court and government. It is sometimes difficult for those outside the service to determine whether the function now is a servant of the government of the day, of parliament as a whole, or of the public. Within public health, should the advocacy be for health, through the powers of an employing authority; for health across a wide spectrum, involving influence rather than power; or for the views of the public, which might result in a loss of health advocacy in favour of health care? A public health advocate may find it difficult at times to maintain independence in a corporate NHS unless the roles, the requirements, and the boundaries are clear.

Similarly the role of the representative of the public in corporate decision making may be difficult to combine with the traditional basis for decision making. The opinions of the public health professional and the public may not always be the same, the choice between the two approaches may provide a very different power base from which to operate in a corporate system. As the public health professional takes on the role of activist he or she will be recognised less as a professional with unique skills. Although it may at times help to achieve certain objectives in the short term, it remains to be seen whether it helps to strengthen the profession and its potential influence in the longer term. The challenge in the future may well lie in maintaining the standing of the profession of public health as a discipline which combines professional knowledge and skills of public health with the courage to deal with the right issues.

With the internal market philosophy the management and planning of health services have become more decentralised or even fragmented. This allows an approach in which the services are tailored to the needs of the communities, but it also means that there are many more decision makers with whom the public health practitioners have to work to create optimal services. Under the circumstances it may be difficult to claim attention for health promotion programmes that go beyond the smaller communities and patient populations. The more decentralised approach also allows for and even encourages differentiation, to be viewed positively as community centred priorities but also negatively as creating inequalities in which more powerful constituencies will always do better. A director of public health may then yet again have to be the representative of the interests of the most deprived communities, a corporate player who is not willing to overlook some of the consequences of the new rules of the game. As the common values such as equity are no longer necessarily seen to be the sole basis of the NHS, the trade off between equity and efficiency may not be weighted in the same way by all corporate players or even by the majority of the population served by the NHS.

This dilemma has also been noted in other countries, sometimes even more so in countries that do not have a national health service. In many western countries the combination of an ageing population and a reduction in government spending has reopened the debate on the future of the welfare state. As medical technology evolves and costs of health care continue to rise, some countries are reconsidering the possibility of a two tier system in which some services will be accessible only to those able to pay for them. Those countries that have openly discussed priority setting or basic care packages (such as Sweden and the Netherlands) have done so from a strong public health perspective, but most of the health care reforms introduced in many of these countries have also opened the system to more competitive elements. These market forces may well introduce incentives for efficiency (even if based on risk selection) that will make it hard to maintain an equity perspective. The public health advocate will require considerable skills in such a situation to promote the population perspective effectively and to avoid being marginalised as an old fashioned idealist.

Managing the tensions

As circumstances change the tensions that arise from different public health functions also change. In managing these tensions it seems to be important for a strong profession to take the initiative on the issues to be dealt with in the future, to set the agenda, but also to propose appropriate structural conditions to allow for these functions to be best combined.

Future challenges for public health

The most important aspect of public health practice remains the promotion of the health of the population. This can be done by initiating preventive interventions, by putting forward the population's health perspective in the allocation of resources in the health service, and by trying to influence determinants of health outside the health services. It is in these last two areas that conflicts with corporacy are most likely to emerge, as these are the areas where the vested interests that influence health must be challenged and where consideration must be given even to reallocation of resources from and within health care.

Public health issues are long standing. Successes in areas such as infant mortality and infections ensure survival to the age of chronic disease and disability. New infections, such as HIV, new technologies in the food industry, and escalating pollution are but a few new problems to be tackled through public health measures. In these changing circumstances people with public health skills to analyse health problems and devise solutions will be indispensable in many organisations. Public health practice, however, goes beyond its technical contributions to the advocacy of health promoting policies and the implementation of change.

Although the role of health authorities continues to change, the nature of the contribution of public health professionals to the achievement of corporate goals will probably remain unaltered. The combination of professional influence and capacity as a facilitator of change results in a powerful corporate player. In the future the public health professional may have to deal with some public health issues that so far have been inadequately recognised or even ignored. More than in the past they will also concern a critical evaluation of health services provided for the community.

Public health practitioners need to establish an authoritative agenda for action in the future. The lead may come from the government, through the chief medical officers; from the field, through the directors of public health; from the wider profession through the Faculty of Public Health Medicine or academic departments; or from the public including pressure groups. The range of potentially relevant topics is huge, from specific problems of provision of services with the NHS to the global environment:

- Waiting times
- The closure of hospitals
- Emergency admissions
- Care in the community
- Poor clinical practice
- The implications of a two tier system
- Resource allocation
- Legalisation of cannabis
- Education and nursery vouchers
- Ecological issues.

It is obvious that public health professionals may not be able to tackle all of these topics simultaneously. It is very important, however, for the profession to feel that it is not only reacting to changes in the corporate environment of the new NHS but taking responsibility for putting issues on the political agenda. It must ensure the visibility of subjects which affect the population's health, even if they are not the priorities of the NHS. In deciding on the priority of the subjects to be covered it may be useful to review such topics, considering for each:

- What is the importance for public health?
- Has there been a clearly expressed public health view?
- If so, where did it come from?
- If not, why not?
- Were we afraid—because it is too political or would lose us friends?
- Was it too difficult?
- Was there not enough evidence?
- Was there not enough time?
- Are we inhibited and no one wants to take the lead?
- How could this issue be dealt with from a public health perspective?
- Who should take responsibility?
- If an effective public health view is promulgated will it prejudice corporacy at any level?
- Is it a short term issue that diverts from the overall strategy?

The future of public health

In the past public health professionals have been very influential. The profession is increasingly able to bring together the technical, advocacy, and corporate contributions to promote successful interventions. The environment in which public health practitioners have to function may have changed, the problems to be dealt with may vary, but essentially the functions remain the same. The changing environment will require a flexibility and adaptability which again is not new. In assessing problems in the future, whatever the organisational context, they will need to decide:

- Should we do it?—A value based decision
- Shall we do it?—A decision based on resources and priorities
- How do we do it best?—An evidence based decision.

It is in the first of these decisions that the responsibility of the public health professional in a corporate structure may be most threatened. If an independent assessment of the threats to the population's health is seen to criticise the organisation to which the public health professional belongs, or other vested interests, a corporate player may be silenced. If one truly believes, however, that it is in the best interest of the population's health to have such an advocate, appropriate structural conditions must be created to allow this function to be preserved. The annual report and the continuing independence of the director of public health in presenting it may be the most tangible result of such structural conditions. A question remains, however, about the target audience for the report: is it to inform the top of the NHS, the democratically elected representatives, or the public?

Before 1974 one could argue that there was some legitimacy in that the medical officer of health was the agent of a local authority and answerable to a health committee of democratically elected councillors. Since then, the democratic deficit in the NHS at local level may have changed the nature of public health responsibility. It is certainly not clear, however, that the introduction of elected health authority members would necessarily lead to greater legitimacy for public health measures.

If it is essential in any health system to have at least an independent director of public health to voice what is best for the population's health, potential conflicts between the advocacy role and the corporate identity have to be accepted. One way out of this dilemma might be for the NHS, rather than the director only, to make it very clear that it wants to maintain this public health advocacy function and to provide the safeguards necessary for this function to be fulfilled. This will ultimately strengthen the way in which the NHS is seen to care about the population's health.

The Partner:

The Royal College of Physicians of Edinburgh

The Question:

What should be the freedoms and constraints of medical professionalism in the context of managed healthcare?

The Writer:

Dr Graham Buckley, Director, Scottish Council for Postgraduate Medical and Dental Education, Edinburgh

Think Tank Members:

Mr TEW Brett, Chief Executive, Dundee Hospitals NHS Trust
Mrs Dorothy Burns-Brown, Surgical Ward Sister, Royal Infirmary of Edinburgh NHS Trust
Dr Margaret Cook, Consultant Haematologist, St John's Hospital at Howden NHS Trust
Dr Colin Currie, Consultant Geriatrician, Royal Infirmary of Edinburgh NHS Trust
Dr Ian Laing, Consultant Neonatologist and Clinical Director, Royal Infirmary of Edinburgh NHS Trust
The Very Reverend Dr WJG McDonald, Former Parish Minister and Moderator of the General Assembly of the Church of Scotland
Professor Sheila McLean, International Bar Association Professor of Law and Ethics in Medicine, University of Glasgow
Mr Malcolm McNicol, Consultant Orthopaedic Surgeon, Royal Infirmary of Edinburgh NHS Trust
Professor Marshall Marinker, Visiting Professor of General Practice, UMDS, London and Advisor in Health Care Policy and Medical Education, MSD Ltd
Mr David Nicholson, Chartered Accountant, Managing Partner, KPMG, Edinburgh and President, Edinburgh Chamber of Commerce
Dr Tony Toft (Chair), Consultant Physician, Royal Infirmary of Edinburgh NHS Trust

3 The limits of professional freedom

GRAHAM BUCKLEY

Life is short
The art long
Opportunity fleeting
Experiment treacherous
Judgment difficult

HIPPOCRATES: *Aphorisms 1*

Introduction

Almost every week medicine is in the headlines. The lack of an intensive care bed for a sick patient, the prospect of a major advance in treatment against cancer, or the latest developments in imaging techniques quickly captures the public attention and becomes news. More often, news is made because of conflict. On the surface, disputes may seem to be about poor administration resulting in the closure of hospital wards or repeated delays in scheduling the operation for a patient. Behind the detail of the particular problem lies a basic fact in all developed countries: the technical capability for delivering effective health care has outstripped the will and capacity of societies collectively to provide the resources to meet personal expectations. The management of limited resources inevitably results in priority setting and rationing. The astonishing technical advances of the past 50 years have raised expectations of improved health and dramatically increased the costs of health care. These have made medicine politically sensitive and increased the potential for conflict between the profession, politicians, and the public. Politicians demand better value for money and perceive an unfettered medical profession as a profligate spender. They see the need to contain and constrain doctors within a managed and regulated environment. The current climate in medicine is one of distinct unease, in which the profession sees its value system and ethical basis to be under attack. This chapter explores that value system and how old ethics can deal with the problems of the new medicine.

The tale of the taxi driver

> "Where are you off to? A medical meeting? You a doctor? Great bunch but what's going on? I had this right hip done beautifully by the professor three years ago. Lovely job—part of a trial apparently. No delay and a special alloy individually made for me. No trouble since but the left hip soon started playing up. Went to the GP who said that the trial was over and because the practice was now fundholding I had to be referred to the local hospital and not to the professor. Apparently this would be at least £2000 cheaper than trying to send me back to the professor who might not see me anyway. Been on a waiting list for a year—couldn't work because of the stiffness and pain. Being self employed I've lost a lot of money. The end result is OK but not as good as the right hip. Technically I guess all the doctors did their jobs well but I just don't think it was a very professional way of dealing with my problem."

There is nothing unusual about this story, which was related to me on my way to one of the panel meetings set up to consider the question posed at the head of this chapter. It does illustrate current complexities and constraints in the practice of medicine and stimulated discussion about the nature of professionalism and the ethical basis of the practice of medicine:

- Does continuing responsibility for a patient end when the research trial is complete?
- Is the benefit of a research study for the doctor, the patient, or the greater good?
- Should financial considerations influence treatment decisions?; If so, by whom and how should decisions be made?
- Should the impact of disability on the patient's finances (earning capacity, hidden costs of informal care) influence priority for treatment—that is, queue jumping?

The panel considering these questions consisted mainly of doctors leavened by representatives of other professions; nursing, law, accountancy, and the church.

Professionalism

At the heart of any consideration of professionalism is a paradox. The view from within a profession emphasises positive attributes. For example, the report of the meeting on core values for the medical profession, held by the BMA at the end of 1994, gave emphasis to "ancient virtues distilled over time". These ancient virtues were considered to include commitment, caring, compassion, integrity, competence, spirit of inquiry, confidentiality, responsibility, and advocacy.

These attributes make up the altruistic ideal of what it is to be a member of a profession. For all professions there is the generally accepted concept that a professional person has a duty of care to a client or patient which goes beyond contractual responsibilities pertaining in commercial transactions. This duty of care is so well established as to be understood in the legal sense. Failures in duty of care can result in civil actions for accountants and lawyers as well as for doctors.

There are negative aspects of professionalism. Sociologists think of professions in terms of power and privilege. Power can be misused and privilege exploited for personal gain. Economists use the term "thin trading" to describe transactions where the customer has limited knowledge about the quality of the service being provided. The customer/consumer/patient gains reassurance if the service is provided by a professional person as this implies long training with defined standards of behaviour and skills assured through robust self regulation. This ideal is not always achieved, and the privilege of providing a monopoly service can engender complacency and authoritarianism. Self interest rather than service may be the motivation in the procedures adopted by profession.

The paradox between altruism and self interest is more keenly felt in medicine than in other professions. Accountants and lawyers do not have altruism as a prominent badge on their collective corporate cloaks. Altruism in medicine comes from its identification as a vocation. The direct intervention of doctors in the fundamentals of life, death, and suffering have given and continue to give doctors a special place in society. In earlier societies medicine and religion were intimately interrelated. The doctor as magus or shaman was a central figure in all primitive societies. The magical powers of doctors and medicine have been enhanced rather than weakened through the marvels of biotechnology and medical science.

Looking to the future, doctors need to have a vision of themselves which can encompass ancient virtues and legitimate self interest. This can be achieved if the profession is able to examine its ethical base openly and honestly. The polarity of much current debate between doctors and managers derives from untested beliefs that different value systems are being used by the two groups. Before examining these beliefs, I will use a brief history of medicine to seek insights from the past as to how our ethical traditions have developed in the face of expanding capabilities and cultural shifts.

The Hippocratic tradition

It is not necessary to be conscious of a tradition to be influenced by it. The principles of the school of medicine at Cos and the Hippocratic oath shape present day relationships between doctors and patients and between doctors and managers. The behaviour of doctors, managers, and patients is not a simple reaction to immediate problems. Each party brings to an encounter unstated but powerful expectations, assumptions, and patterns of behaviour that are an amalgam of the personal and collective experiences which make up our culture.

The principles and the oath ascribed to Hippocrates are the starting point in this ethical journey through the history of medicine and serve as a guide to the ethical dilemmas modern medicine has created and seeks to tackle. In some respects, emphasis on the Hippocratic tradition is the result of a successful nineteenth-century public relations promotion aimed at gaining professional status for doctors through the 1858 Medicine Act. Nevertheless, the oath does have continuing relevance and meaning for doctors and patients.

In its compendium of guidance booklets on the *Duties of a Doctor* the General Medical Council (GMC) does not cite Hippocrates in relation to the principles it enunciates, but they are in large measure paraphrased elements of the oath:

- Make the care of your patient your first concern
- Treat every patient politely and considerately
- Respect a patient's dignity and privacy

- Listen to patients and respect their views
- Give patients information in a way they can understand
- Respect the rights of patients to be fully informed about decisions about their care
- Keep your professional knowledge and skills up to date
- Recognise the limits of your professional competence
- Be honest and trustworthy
- Respect and protect confidential information
- Make sure that your personal beliefs do not prejudice your patients' care
- Act quickly to protect patients from risk if you have good reason to believe that you or a colleague may not be fit to practise
- Avoid abusing your position as a doctor
- Work with colleagues in the ways that best serve patients' interests.

Apart from some additional references to proscribing the use of the knife, forbidding sexual commerce with women in the household of the sick, and the initial homage given to Apollo, the oath covers most of the principles listed above. In addition, the oath places the relationship between student and teacher at the centre of the practice of medicine. This is a sad omission from the GMC's list. The terms doctor and professor both derive from teaching, their original meanings being retained in the universities. Professors, as distinct from doctors, were the people who were paid to teach. The rich array of meanings we give to professional and professionalism derive from this origin. A professional is someone who has rare knowledge and skills but is also trading on these for money. As well as denoting high levels of commitment and competence, the term professional has also acquired the meaning of calculated and cynical breaking of rules to protect self interest, as in the professional foul in association football. The term profession is therefore a snare and a trap. It can mean too many different things. It may provide a false sense of security in implying that a shared set of principles and values defines the profession.

If we confine ourselves to the clinical encounter the ethical strand which leads from Hippocrates to the present day is intact and affords a beneficial shared trust between patients and doctors. The consultation is at the heart of medicine but is not the whole of medicine. The Hippocratic oath and the GMC's list of principles naturally focus on the care of the individual patient. In the statement "act quickly to protect patients from risk if you have reason to believe that you or a colleague may not be fit to practise", the GMC has moved slowly and painfully to insist that doctors carry corporate responsibility for their colleagues.

For centuries all doctors could feel comfortable with the general ethical principal of beneficence. Even here technical advance has created ethical problems. Should medicine strive to do everything that it is competent to do? Is the principle of beneficence upheld by giving antibiotics to treat bronchopneumonia in a severely demented, bed bound elderly patient? It is the ethical principles of justice and equity, however, that pose most problems for doctors. Pellegrino regards competence, integrity, and compassion as first order medical ethical responsibilities, relating, as they do, to the individual. He suggests that doctors have a leading role with regard to equity and utility in health care, but this does not carry the same imperative as first order responsibilities. Finally, he considers that there are third order ethical responsibilities which doctors uphold simply as citizens. This analysis by Pellegrino is attractive. It allows the doctor to retain the role of advocacy for the patient while as a collective venture with colleagues attempting to define what the principles of justice and equity mean in determining access to care.

Can valid distinction be drawn in the way that Pellegrino does between first and second order ethical responsibilities? Such an approach assumes the primacy of the individual above the group and requires the doctor to afford the individual such primacy. Advances in medicine since the early nineteenth-century have questioned this basic premise. An early attempt to tackle the issue was by Thomas Percival in his book *Medical Ethics* published in 1803. This book was stimulated by the development of the infirmary and pays as much attention to etiquette as it does to ethics. Percival attempted to sort out problems of precedence between practitioners in an era when doctors were starting to work together for the first time. The increasingly corporate nature of medicine and the increasing understanding of public health medicine in the nineteenth-century was reflected in the prodigious work of Jeremy Bentham in promoting all kinds of social reforms for the greater good. This utilitarian principle articulated by John Stuart Mill is undeniably a first order ethical responsibility for politicians and health service managers.

We have arrived at the heart of the problem. Doctors, especially those with clinical responsibilities because of their direct involvement with the suffering and needs of individual patients, naturally regard the principle of beneficence, to use Pellegrino's terminology, as a first order ethical responsibility. This carries with it respect for patient autonomy and a requirement for the doctor to be competent and to act on behalf of the patient as an advocate for the use of health resources. Managers, on the other hand, must give primacy to the principles of equity and justice, seeking to follow the utilitarian principle of the greatest good for the greatest number. Before looking at some examples of how these principles may be in conflict in different parts of the health service, consideration needs to be given to what is meant by management and who are the managers in the NHS.

Management

The plethora of books on management on sale in airports offers an intriguing insight into the nature of the modern world. The titles, style, and substance of the management books by the latest gurus and prophets seem to offer a tantalising glimpse of the holy grail to managers in transit from dealing with one crisis to making a new crisis at their destination. Management, like general practice, defies definition. It can be characterised and many of its characteristics are shared with general practice: uncertainty, adaptability, and an absence of fixed boundaries. Much more fruitful than attempts to define management is to describe what managers do. Popper has pointed out that this is the most valuable form of definition. There is no essence of management only a knowledge base, a range of skills, and, often unstated but always present, a set of values which determine the way in which knowledge and skills are used. The knowledge base for managers varies considerably depending on the context in which they operate. It is the values and skills which provide a measure of unity. Efficiency and effectiveness—pursuit of the utilitarian principle of achieving the greater good—is the dominant aim for managers working in the public services. The pre-eminent skill of a manager is the ability to work with and through others in achieving this aim.

The NHS

The main impression gained from visiting doctors in other countries is the similarity of the agenda for change in health care. The drivers of change discussed elsewhere in this book are international in their impact: demographic shifts, information technology, and the increasing expectations for biotechnology and medicine to be effective in extending the quantity and quality of life. The responses to these pressures for change are also similar beneath the surface structures of particular systems of health care and social security. Even in the most liberal insurance based health care systems there is the desire to strengthen primary care and self care as a means of restraining the rising costs of secondary and tertiary care.

Of direct relevance to the theme of this chapter is the growing insistence by governments and other insurers to measure outcomes of care and the effectiveness of treatment in terms of value for money. This is the language of managers and politicians, and these groups share a common purpose in seeking to deliver more from a finite level of resource. Not surprisingly, doctors, as a major element of that resource, feel pressured to work longer and more intensively to achieve externally imposed targets. Again in the language of management, their productivity is under scrutiny. Part of the resistance exhibited by doctors to being managed stems from a sense that the easily measurable is not necessarily the most important indicator of quality and health care. Clinical decision making is complex, and doctors resist and resent the application of production line concepts to health care.

The battle lines between doctors and managers in the United Kingdom have their roots in the extraordinary nature and history of the NHS. To understand the current issues and conflicts in health care in this country, an appreciation of the development of the NHS is required. As all embracing and pervasive as the weather, the NHS is so embedded in the national culture that, like the weather, everybody complains about it but nobody questions its existence. In its complexities it also resembles the weather as an example of the fashionable mathematical model of deterministic chaos, in which patterns can be discerned but prediction is uncertain.

The key features of the NHS have been present since its inception in 1948: comprehensive in its demographic, geographic, and service coverage; free at the point of use; a protected position for general practitioners as gatekeepers to other services; the rigid separation of primary and secondary care; reasonable equity in the distribution of resources. Despite recent rises in costs, the NHS remains in comparative terms remarkably good value and for the past 50 years it has been a solid bulwark of socialism amid the swirling changes of privatisation and competition.

It is interesting to look back at the reactions of the medical profession to the introduction of the NHS. As with almost all major reforms in the organisation of health care, the profession collectively opposed its implementation initially, although many doctors individually contributed to the planning process. The battle cry of opposition was the perceived threat to clinical freedom from the introduction of socialised medicine. Salutary to note, the successful method used to overcome opposition was to provide financial incentives for the group of doctors considered by the government to be most influential. The lesson was well learned by politicians, and the technique has been used regularly since to induce changes in behaviour by doctors.

The early years of the NHS were characterised by administration rather than management. Important decisions continued to be taken by doctors within the overall resources made available by the government. Medical superintendents and matrons ruled the hospital supported by administrators who knew their place within the hierarchy. The NHS was a mirror of a deferential society in which "the doctor knew best". As in its tolerance of mediocre restaurants, the general public was willing in the aftermath of the second world war to accept basic levels of service with no frills and complied with rationing in the form of long waiting lists for treatment.

The cracks in the paternalistic structure began to appear in the 1960s. The youth revolution of 1968 put paid to much of the automatic deference previously given to those in authority. The oil crisis of the early 1970s brought severe pressure on resources for all forms of public service including health. At the same time, reports such as *Sans Teeth, Sans Everything* identified the failure of the health service to cater for the needs of the elderly and the mentally ill. The response was to introduce consensus management to try to achieve a more equitable distribution of resources. This was tacit recognition that previous decision making was often heavily influenced by high profile, charismatic doctors pursuing their own particular enthusiams. Consensus management in retrospect was the first of the checks on the power of the medical profession within the NHS. It was weak and bureaucratic and led to a rapid increase in the number of administrators. It was also criticised at the time for failing to take the hard decisions, producing a service paralysed by fudge and compromise.

The scene was set for Sir Roy Griffiths and his inquiry into the organisation of the NHS. He based his review around the question, Is anybody in charge? The simple answer was "No", and he saw the need for general managers responsible for the overall *performance* of the operational units within the NHS. Performance is a key word which has a different resonance for doctors and managers. For doctors, performance means achieving excellence in the care of individual patients, whereas the term for managers suggests gaining maximum output for a given level of resource. The acceptance by the government of the Griffiths report in 1984 had much greater impact on the management of health care in the United Kingdom than any other change over the past 50 years. It established the managers rather than doctors as the prime decision makers in the use of resources. The reforms of 1990 merely separated two sets of managers to clarify their roles and increase their accountability.

Historically, the medical profession has been slow to respond to change and easy to manipulate through exploitation of divisions within the profession. Only now, 10 years after the introduction of general management, are doctors, in significant numbers, learning to use and incorporate the techniques of management to achieve their objectives. There are signs that some doctors are moving on to a new agenda after a decade of retreat and complaint. The next section will examine some of the intriguing ways in which doctors are engaged in and with management.

Medical directors and clinical directors

The dichotomy between medicine and management in the minds of doctors is clearly visible when attempts are made to recruit a new medical director or clinical director of an NHS trust. The general lack of enthusiasm is expressed in terms of becoming one of "them" or joining the "enemy". Some of the antipathy to managers and management is breaking down through the effectiveness of some pioneering medical directors. Still, the route from consultant to medical director is seen within the profession as a sideways step at best rather than a career progression. In any other organisation the move from operational activity to a managerial position is seen as normal advancement. The fact that this is not the case in the NHS perpetuates a fault line which is detrimental. Some of the gulf between doctors and managers stems from the different sets of responsibilities discharged by the two groups. Independent of any resource constraints, doctors remain individually professionally accountable for the level of care provided to a patient. The NHS trust carries medical indemnity insurance but alone the doctor is accountable to the GMC. Managers, on the other hand, are accountable for their use of resources. Their job security is at risk if their efficiency and effectiveness are found wanting. Jibes about performance related pay for managers and rejoinders about distinction awards for doctors serve not to demonstrate basic human similarities in the desire for recognition and reward but reinforce perceived differences in culture. Given this background, it is not surprising that medical directors find it difficult to bridge the divide in contributing effectively as part of the senior management team while also providing leadership for the doctors working in a trust.

Leadership of the functional units within a trust has usually been vested in a senior clinician, the managerial responsibilities denoted by the title clinical director. In most trusts, clinical directors have simply been given the poisoned chalice drunk by many middle managers—responsibility without power. The motivation of many clinical directors in accepting these posts seems to be defensive. They hope for early access to information about policy shifts in the belief that this will limit damage to their range of services from the demands of senior management.

The solution to the problems outlined above must be through establishing mutual respect between doctors and managers. This will be helped by greater honesty and improved clarity about the roles expected of doctors and managers. Is the doctor on a trust board a senior manager or the representative of shopfloor workers? Ambiguities about the role of medical directors could be resolved if doctors become chief executives. In retrospect, the present era may come to be seen as a curious interlude in which it was assumed that managerial skills acquired in the monoculture of industry could be transplanted successfully into the health service jungle. Time will tell whether doctors are willing to become managers and whether doctors will be more amenable to being managed by other doctors rather than by general managers. History suggests that they will be.

GP fundholding

Nothing in the 1990 NHS reforms created more controversy than the introduction of GP fundholding. It continues to divide the general practice community, the rhetoric of confrontation referring to ethics and beliefs rather than a debate about the measured effects of introducing fundholding. GPs and their antecedents—the apothecaries, barber surgeons, and country doctors—have always managed their own businesses. The independent contractor status of GPs within the NHS continues this basic pattern: they employ staff and have regard to expenditure as well as income in judging the performance of the business in providing good care for individual patients and for the practice population.

What is the fundamental difference between fundholding and non-fundholding practices for this innovation to have created such a furore? Fundholding in its different forms provides GPs with a budget to buy services on behalf of their patients. These services are those which the practice provide itself as part of contractually defined General Medical Services. Fundholding GPs are therefore both purchasers and providers. The care of patients in primary care is determined by the efficiency and effectiveness of the practice in managing its own services. Is this different from the management skills required to purchase services effectively from other health care providers? Some doctors do think that there is a difference because of the huge discrepancy in costs between primary and secondary care. These doctors think that the GP's role as advocate for the patient is weakened by knowledge that referral for expensive treatment will considerably impact on the budget. The budget managed by fundholding GPs is finite, and incentives are offered to encourage underspending. Critics of the system claim that the fundholding GP cannot act as both advocate and jury.

The counterargument accepts that the potential for conflict exists within fundholding practices but points out that conflict between advocacy and rationing has always been present within the NHS. Previously it has been masked by impersonal devices such as waiting lists and quotas for expensive operations or treatments determined by people remote from the clinical interaction and thus unable to appreciate the weight of the particular needs of individual patients. Fundholders claim that they are in the best position to bring clinical and managerial skills together to act in the interest of patients in providing high quality primary care and shaping secondary care.

In fundholding much rests on the personal skills of the general practitioner manager. Not surprisingly, the audit commission report published in May 1996 showed that in this, as in other attributes, GPs exhibit a wide range of skills and competencies in the use they make of fundholding opportunities. Some fundholders have, through energy, imagination, and negotiation, stimulated and tailored secondary care for the benefit of their patients. Others have made no effective use of their new opportunities and have consumed resources through the additional administration needed to operate the system. At least the debate is now moving on from fundamentalist confrontations between protagonists and opponents to a consideration of the available evidence of the effects of the reforms. Individual doctors are able to be creative in making contracts in ways that manage to combine personal and corporate ethics: for example, fundholding practices recycling the savings they achieve for the benefit of all practices in a locality. This indicates how black and white views on the ethical aspects of the scheme can become blurred when doctors show a commitment to striving not only for improvements in health care for their own patients but extend this to a concern for the whole population. In the main, however, there is still a divide within general practice regarding fundholding. The divide is a reflection of more general political leanings and beliefs. Stated in bald terms, it is the question of whether we believe society is best served through promotion of personal freedom or through collective action. With a democratic deficit within health care, personal freedom and collective action in the Health Service tends to mean doctors rather than patients.

Fundholding has been actively promoted by government as a way of both containing costs and creating a primary care led NHS. With little external support collectively minded GPs have produced alternative models to fundholding while sharing the same objectives. The creation of these locality groups demonstrates that financial inducement is not the only motivation for doctors to take on managerial responsibilities and money not the only resource. Time and skill are resources which have at least as much impact as money in determining the quality of care in general practice. Effective practices are those in which the importance of these non-monetary resources are recognised and managed. Do the right patients see the right professionals at the right time? Does the practice have the appropriate range of skills to make the most effective use of time? A highly successful distance learning course for GPs in the 1980s was entitled *If Only I Had The Time?* Thousands of GPs participated in the course, which made management palatable because it highlighted the key importance of time management.

Innovative contracting

The Orwellian use of language is a feature in the modern NHS. The term "NHS Trust" did not instantly engender trust. Trust, like respect, is earned not imposed. Innovative contracting as a label sounds positive and promising. Decoded, it means "privately managed health care within the NHS". Health authorities and fundholders are being asked to explore and agree contracts with pharmaceutical companies and others to provide total packages of care for defined groups of patients. As an example, people with insulin dependent diabetes could be offered all their specialist care by a company which produces insulin. Doctors and nurses seeing the patients would be paid for by the pharmaceutical company, and, naturally, the company's own range of drugs would be considered first in formulating the treatment plans.

In the United Kingdom, managed health care, of the type outlined above, has received encouragement only for exploration from the Department of Health. As yet, no permission has actually been given to sign contracts with private suppliers of care. As with many other innovations in the NHS in recent years this form of contracting originates and has already been tried out in the United States.

The fact that this form of providing care is even being considered is a testimony to the perceived power and effectiveness of managers. What the pharmaceutical company is really selling to the NHS is the prospect of more efficient management. Just as Sir Roy Griffiths assumed that general managers from industry could operate successfully within the NHS, the assumption made in considering privately managed care is that the management systems, which have made pharmaceutical companies successful, will translate readily into the successful management of health care. Utilising the companies' management skills and systems in the provision of health care is claimed to contain cost and guarantee high quality. The fact that the pharmaceutical companies are in business to make profits is not apparently an issue. After all, other hospital services such as catering, cleaning, and laboratory services have been privatised so why not patient care? Is the doctor or nurse employed by the pharmaceutical company in any way different from the partners from within a fundholding general practice. Each of the professionals working in these environments could feel financial pressure to choose one product over another or pursue one line of treatment over another. Within each of these structures the patient is dependent on the professional integrity of the doctor to give the best possible advice, independent of any cost considerations. The difference between present contracting arrangements and the type of innovative contracting described above is that savings accruing from efficiencies are retained in the health service in the former but become profits for share holders in the latter.

Many doctors will find it extraordinary that the health service should be even considering commercial management of health care. The evidence so far from contracted-out services is that they can be provided more cheaply but have an adverse impact on the integration of care and team work. It is not a major consideration when the services concerned are not central or crucial for patient care. If clinical care is contracted out to private suppliers and direct responsibility for the patient handed over to a commercial company has the heart of the NHS been removed? In posing this question, am I providing yet another example of a reactionary doctor resisting an exciting innovation which offers more for patients than the traditional systems provided by the NHS. I think not.

The issue concerns the obligations of a public service. Just as a profession is defined by a duty of care so is a public service. The duty of care is not limited by contract. Will a private company continue to provide a service to the patient who unexpectedly develops a new disease? Not if it is omitted from the contract. A public service will be obliged to continue to provide care. Comprehensiveness does not come cheap, and managed care contracts will be likely to have the same small print exclusions as private health insurance so that the major financial risks continue to be borne by the NHS rather than the company.

The concept of privately managed health care should be the final spur for doctors to realise that management is too important to be left to managers.

Humanities are the hormones

I began this chapter by indicating that medicine is a conflict zone. Within health care the conflict is experienced most commonly between doctors and managers. The sources of the conflict which reside in the ethical basis of medicine and management have been explored. Characteristics of the tensions between doctors and managers in the United Kingdom have been described in the context of the development, reforms, and innovation which have occurred in the NHS. Looking to the future, the potential for continuing conflict is all too apparent. Technology will make it possible to do more and more for people at ever rising costs. What are the limits to clinical freedom and who should determine them? The key question concerns not the freedoms and constraints of doctors in the context of managed health care, but rather the freedoms and constraints of patients within the NHS.

The technical advances in medicine have made it clear that there can be no fixed answer. Constraints, conflicts, and tensions will continue in the health arena. Questions surrounding euthanasia, the rights of unborn children, genetic manipulation, and organ transplantation have to be dealt with on a broad front. Philosophy, politics, sociology, and theology as well as medicine have valuable contributions to make. Even more broadly, we need the humanities to help us understand the nature of the issues themselves. What is meant by quality of life? Is it purely a personal notion or one that has some shared meaning? Medical science has not much to offer in determining the answer, and yet it is an important question when seeking ways to determine distribution of resources in an equitable way.

Medical education is deficient in the humanities. Although the reforms in undergraduate education are providing new opportunities; science and the acquisition of technical skills has largely driven the humanities from the medical curriculum. Without an appreciation about the history of ideas or a framework for analysing the values used in clinical decisions, doctors can become mere technicians, unaware of the effects that their own prejudices have on their own clinical work. In his book *The New Medicine and the Old Ethics*, Jonsen refers to the lecture given by Sir William Osler to the British Classical Society in 1919, when he used the phrase "humanities are the hormones" to emphasise the power of the humanities to lubricate and energise society. The special study modules in the new undergraduate curriculum provide a splendid opportunity to reintroduce the humanities into medicine so that medical students acquire the hormones of history, philosophy, and ethics. Grounding in these disciplines is needed if doctors are to contribute to the continuing public debates on health care necessary in an open society.

The title of the chapter refers to a power struggle which is taking place between doctors and managers within the NHS. The real issue, however, is whether these two powerful groups, together with politicians, can honestly engage with the public in assessing the opportunities, risks, and demands that modern medicine presents. This is an educational agenda. Warnock writes of education as the transfer of values from one generation to another and sees education as a means for understanding the narrative within which we exist. Doctors, managers, and patients can, through education, respect the contribution each group can make in making health care humane as well as efficient and make the next page in the narrative one which our children can enjoy.

Further reading

Anonymous. Medicine in conflict (editorial). *Proceedings of the Royal College of Physicians of Edinburgh* 1995;**25**:539–41.

Audit Commission. *What the doctor ordered.* London: 1996, HMSO.

Beecher HK. Ethics and clinical research. *N Engl J Med* 1966;**74**:1354–60.

British Medical Association. *Core values for the medical profession.* London: BMJ Publishing, 1994.

Bunker JP. Can professionalism service the market place? *BMJ* 1994;**308**: 1179–80.

General Medical Council. *Duties of a doctor.* London: GMC, 1995.

Griffiths P. *Beyond management.* London: Institute of Health Service Management, 1996.

Harrison S. *Managing the NHS: shifting the frontier?* London: Chapman Hall, 1988.

Jonsen AR. *The new medicine and the old ethics.* Cambridge, Massachusetts: Harvard University Press, 1990.

MacIntyre A. Medicine as bureaucracy. In: Cassell EJ, Siegler M, eds. *Changing values in medicine.* New York: University Publications of America, 1979.

Pellegrino ED. Missing dimensions in hippocratic ethics. In: Bulger RJ, ed. *Hippocrates revisited: a search for meaning.* New York: Medcom Press, 1973.

Rothman DJ. *Strangers at the bedside: a history of how law and bio-ethics transformed medical decision making.* New York: Basic Books, 1991.

Simpson J, Smith R. *Management for doctors.* London: BMJ Publishing, 1995.
Thompson AE. A corporate approach to ethics in medicine. In: Phillips CI, ed. *Logic in medicine.* 2nd ed. London: BMJ Publishing, 1995.
Turner BS. *Medical power and social knowledge.* London: Sage, 1987.
Warnock M. *Imagination and time.* Oxford: Blackwell, 1994.
Weir A, Geyer-Kordesch, French R. *Doctors and ethics: the earlier setting of professional ethics.* Amsterdam: Rodopi, 1993.

The Partner:

The Royal College of General Practitioners

The Question:

How can 'Evidence Based Medicine' help patients in general practice?

The Writer:

Dr Kieran Sweeney, General Practitioner, Exeter

Think Tank Members:

Dr Graham Buckley, Director, Scottish Council for Postgraduate Medical and Dental Education, Edinburgh
Dr Bruce Charlton, Lecturer, Department of Psychology, University of Newcastle
Dr Keith Donaldson, General Practitioner, Edinburgh
Dr Iona Heath, General Practitioner, Kentish Town, London
Professor Roger Jones, Wolfson Professor of General Practice, UMDS
Professor Marshall Marinker, Visiting Professor of General Practice, UMDS, London and Advisor in Health Care Policy and Medical Education, MSD Ltd
Professor Mike Pringle, Professor of General Practice, Nottingham
Dr Bill Reith, Regional Advisor in General Practice, North East Scotland, RCGP Honorary Secretary of Council
Professor Lesley Southgate, Professor of Primary Care and Medical Education
Dr Ben Sweeney, General Practitioner, Glasgow, Chairman, Committee of Medical Ethics RCGP

4 Evidence and uncertainty

KIERAN SWEENEY

GPs act as interpreters of their patients' stories, guardians against the overmedicalisation of their problems, and witnesses to their suffering. Often they must carry out these tasks when the evidence for diagnosis and rational treatment is unavailable, absent, or exhausted. Evidence Based Medicine (EBM) is an approach to clinical problem solving which applies the best, relevant evidence from research to answer clinical questions. It is designed to help doctors perform the rational task of making a diagnosis better on the basis of firm criteria and choosing the proved best treatment. But the method was never intended to apply to situations when there is no firm "evidence". Here doctors must rely on logic, intuition and experience—often regarded with disdain by the proponents of EBM. In summary, EBM is clearly a necessary but not in itself a sufficient condition for the practice of good medicine in primary care. This is the proposition set out in this chapter.

Introduction

The method is described as having five steps.[1–5]

- A clear clinical question is formulated from the patient's presenting problem
- A literature search is carried out to identify relevant published articles which deal with the problem
- The evidence is accessed and evaluated (or critically appraised)
- Valid and useful findings are implemented into clinical practice
- An audit of performance is carried out.

This chapter is divided into four sections. In the first, the principles of EBM are explained and placed in their historical context. The method is clear and appealing and has been enthusiastically received by some general practitioners.[6] But a description of the method[4] and a recent example of its application in an acute medical unit of a teaching hospital[7] were quite heavily criticised in the correspondence columns of the peer reviewed journals in which they appeared. In the second section these criticisms are explored and their justification considered.

The third section describes the nature of general practice. Here, the wide variety of problems that patients present to general practitioners is described and the way that doctors in primary care respond to them. The intention is to examine how best to integrate EBM into the present framework of general practice.

Finally the question, How can patients in general practice benefit from EBM? is covered. The conclusion reached is that GPs have a responsibility to accommodate EBM as a desirable feature of good practice. Patients have a right to receive medical opinions based, when possible, on the best available evidence. But in general practice "the best available evidence" includes a broader concept of relevance and validity than is presently accommodated by the theory and practice of EBM.

Principles

The instigators of EBM claimed that it "aimed to de-emphasise unsystematic clinical experience and intuition as sufficient grounds for taking decisions in clinical practice".[1] Rather the appraisal of evidence from clinical research was to be seen as the evident and proper basis for making decisions about clinical problems. The process can be summarised as follows: patients present with problems which are turned into clinical questions; the answers to these questions are then based on the best available evidence obtained by searching for and critically appraising the relevant studies.

After the description of the method was published[1] a series of articles in the *Journal of the American Medical Association* (*JAMA*) entitled "The users' guide to medical literature" illustrated the principles of EBM in greater detail.[8] The articles explained the basis of the critical appraisal of new information. A major contribution of the series was to demonstrate the calculations and significance of four basic outcome statistics: risk ratios, relative risk reductions (the complement of the risk ratio expressed as a percentage), the calculation of absolute risk reduction, and, finally, the idea of numbers needed to treat (the inverse of the absolute risk). What, then, were the advantages that EBM offered?

Firstly, it offered the possibility of greater efficiency by identifying which treatments or clinical approaches could be usefully incorporated into practice and which could be excluded. Secondly, as a consequence of this, improvements in the quality of decisions about purchasing could be made. Thirdly, the construction of a common language for critical appraisal of new evidence could be developed, which in turn might encourage the design of better trials. Finally, EBM could provide a sound grounding for undergraduate and continuing postgraduate education.

EBM also offered other possibilities. Its principles could be acquired by health care professionals from different backgrounds (including non-clinicians) at any stage of their careers. For example, the Critical Appraisal Skills for Purchasers project, in the former Oxford region, entailed teaching the principles of EBM to purchasers who had no medical training. Ultimately, it is argued, its teaching can extend to consumer groups.[4]

There are, however, daunting problems in attempting to apply the principle of seeking best evidence from research de novo and in relation to each new individual clinical problem. It is conservatively estimated that it would require two hours to focus on a clinical question and then find, appraise, and act on the evidence.[4] It would also require an expensive infrastructure—for example, computer software and access to the Internet. Furthermore, acquiring the necessary skills would necessitate dedicated protected time for postgraduate study. The impracticability of acquiring and applying the time and skills to each clinical problem explains the need to present the fruits of EBM in synopsis form as protocols or guidelines. To date it is the status, validity, and applicability of these synopses (protocols and guidelines) that have been the focus of criticism.

Dawes was one of the first to promote the potential of EBM in general practice.[6] He identified three arguments against its acceptability and put forward a number of counterarguments.

Firstly, some GPs could argue that only a fraction of the medicine practised in general practice has been evaluated in proper trials. Dawes responds to this concern by pointing out that many of the clinical problems encountered by GPs have been the subject of randomised controlled trials but published in specialist journals not regularly read by them. Secondly, hard pressed GPs may be dissuaded from tracking down the evidence because of lack of time. Dawes argues that the introduction of the journal *EBM* will help by collating what the publishers consider to be the best available articles from current peer reviewed journals. The third barrier is that many GPs lack the skills to apply the information offered by EBM, but increasingly courses and workshops on the method are now available. Dawes summarises optimistically thus: "The future is here now; it just isn't evenly distributed yet".[6]

Applications

Two examples of EBM in NHS clinical practice illustrate its application. Over one hundred acute medical admissions were studied to ascertain how many of the treatments that were offered to the patients were evidence based.[7] About 82% of the patients were judged to have received evidence based interventions: 53% had received interventions supported by one or more randomised controlled trials, and 29% were offered interventions unanimously judged to be supported by convincing non-experimental evidence. Similar estimates were arrived at in a study of two days' consecutive consultations in general practice.[9] About 81% of the patients in this study received interventions that were either supported by one or more randomised controlled trials or were supported by convincing but non-experimental evidence.

Reservations

EBM appeals to clinicians because of its perceived clarity of purpose and its attempt to diminish uncertainty. It appeals to managers too, who seek to apply its conclusions to their purchasing decisions. But serious reservations have been expressed.

Iggo challenged the nature of the evidence which forms the basis of EBM: "a major fault with evidence based medicine is its emphasis on randomised controlled trials".[10] Charlton also criticised the heavy reliance on randomised controlled trials (RCTs).[11] He argued that the results of such trials give information only at a population level; such information cannot easily be extrapolated to a particular target group without substantial adjustments based on *contextual* knowledge.

Other concerns have been expressed about the evidential basis of EBM, in particular the use of meta-analysis. It has been argued that the methodology of meta-analysis, which will be considered later in this section, is more arbitrary and subjective than its proponents assert.[12,13] These critics are concerned that, although meta-analysis seems to give a clearer picture of the collated evidence on a particular topic, this clarity may be achieved at the cost of practical judgment, and this presents difficulties when doctors try to apply population evidence to individual patients.

Another critic was clearly angered by some of the claims of EBM.[14] "Evidence based medicine", argued Fowler "is a neologism for informed decision making ... the presumption is made that the practice of medicine was previously based on a direct communication with God or by tossing a coin". Other critics of the same article argued that assignment of diagnoses in this study achieved a reduction in complexity of management at the cost of "drifting from the reality of many patients presenting with more than one problem".[15] These critics also noted that the application of EBM, in this example, excluded "the undiagnosed". This concept will be examined later.

Other criticisms concerned the preoccupation with measuring only what is measurable: "There are no suggestions on how practice relating to unmeasurable aspects is to be guided";[16] and, "Not all that is measured is of value, and not all that is of value can be measured".[15]

A new paradigm?

EBM is a new label but scarcely a new idea. What is innovative, perhaps, is the success of the challenge to doctors about their apparent failure to make consistent use of the best available evidence. Further, it now offers both a strategic and a tactical framework for doing better in this regard in the future.

In the initial exposition of EBM the important and perhaps unsurprising claim made for the approach was that physicians whose practice is based on an understanding of the underlying evidence would provide superior patient care.[1] But was the method so novel as to constitute a paradigm shift—the claim that is now made for it by its proponents?

Kuhn uses the term paradigm to mean a set of shared assumptions or received beliefs in a scientific community. His central thesis was that groups of scientists imagine, think, and research within a cleanly defined set of assumptions which define the possibilities and also the limits of their endeavours—that they use a technical language which encompasses a core group of theories and then occupy themselves largely by solving only those problems that that technical language can express. Only when the need to answer questions that cannot be dealt with within the assumptions of a current paradigm becomes pressing can the assumptions be seriously challenged. Kuhn suggests that it is at (rare) times like these that new paradigms appear. He describes their appearance as "a reconstruction of the field from new fundamentals, a reconstruction that changes some of the most elementary theoretical generalisations".[17]

For decades before the introduction of EBM it had been asserted that such a fundamental paradigm shift was occurring in medicine. In the clinical paradigm that has so dominated medical research in this century, disease was viewed "objectively"—independently from the person who was suffering from it. Mind and body were considered separately, each with its own diseases. The new paradigm which defines the general practice view of medicine "would emphasise the patient, the doctor–patient relationship, and the language of illness".[18]

This holistic paradigm had in fact been part of the research language of clinical medicine for some decades, although compared with the language of a much more powerful twentieth century paradigm, clinical epidemiology, it was relatively muted.

The key contribution to the development of EBM as we know it today was the publication of *Clinical Epidemiology, a Basic Science for Clinical Medicine*,[19] which showed how the principles of clinical epidemiology could be applied to day to day clinical practice.

But the origins of EBM go back further, at least to the 1830s when the Parisian physician PCA Louis developed an epidemiological approach to clinical thinking by comparing the outcomes in two populations of patients offered different treatments.[20] More recent origins of the approach are to be found in the 1960s, when the number of published randomised controlled trials increased exponentially. Their pivotal importance in clinical research was championed by Cochrane, who described the RCT as a "beautiful technique of wide applicability".[21]

Clinical epidemiologists have been working with evidence based approaches for much of the twentieth century.[22] Case-control methods and statistical techniques were developed throughout the first half of the century as sociologists began to tackle health problems as social issues.[23] Doll and Hill were clearly publishing the best available evidence when in 1950 they reported one of the first studies linking smoking and lung cancer.[24]

In general practice, randomised controlled trials began to appear four years after the publication of one as the earliest influential such trials (which compared bed rest and steptomycin in pulmonary tuberculosis); between 1953 and 1991, 90 randomised trials were published in the *British Journal of General Practice*, over three quarters of which had been carried out in primary care.[25]

Evidence based diagnosis

In general practice the concept of "diagnosis" is broader than the strictly biomechanical diagnosis used in RCTs—the cornerstone of the edifice on which the claims of EBM are based. Patients for the most part present their GPs not with diseases but with illnesses—unorganised symptoms and signs. It is from these illnesses that, when appropriate, the doctor reconfigures the narrower concept of the disease.[26] Clearly there are situations when this process of reconfiguration is simple and effective: the patient who consults with a history of increased fluid intake and passing of urine and who is found to have a raised blood sugar concentration of 16 mmols/l is confidently identified as suffering from diabetes. Here, EBM can help to determine the most appropriate method of treatment.

But making a diagnosis is often an evolutionary process. Definitive diagnoses (in this broad sense) may be made retrospectively or indeed not at all. Formulating a diagnosis in general practice can take weeks or months; the exact moment when a diagnosis becomes "clear" may be difficult to determine. Here, the GP uses time appropriately as a powerful diagnostic instrument.[27]

Often, the GP formulates a series of diagnostic hunches early in the consultation, using clues from the doctor's background knowledge of the patient and perhaps the patient's family.[28] Howie distinguishes the diagnostic pathway used in hospital medicine from that used in general practice.[29] He argues that in hospital medicine an analysis of the equal contribution of symptoms, signs, and investigations leads to the formulation of a diagnosis on which treatment decisions are based. This he contrasts with the relative rarity of fully developed diseases in general practice and the frequency with which people present to GPs with symptoms and signs that do not fit established patterns of disease. Hence the GP is forced to bypass confident diagnosis and adopt a decision pathway which approximates to symptomatic treatment.

Learning the diagnostic and decision making skills appropriate to general practice entails a lot of "unlearning" of approaches which have been acquired through medical school education.[30 31] Traditionally diagnosis is taught to medical students (at least initially) as though it were an inductive process—first the facts are gathered without the prejudice of preformed bias, and, only then, when all the relevant pieces of the jigsaw have been assembled, does the full pattern reveal itself.

In fact most clinical problem solving is better taught as a process of hypotheticodeduction[32] or, putting the same idea more simply, "guessing and testing".[33] McWhinney has emphasised some features of decision making in general practice which he believes distinguish it from traditional hypotheticodeductive reasoning.[34] He describes the use of time, probabilities, the importance of the early recognition of disease, and the greater tolerance of uncertainty as central features of decision making in general practice. Willis argues that GPs make use of a complementary intellectual process which leads to the formulation of a diagnosis; he describes this with the telling phrase "intuitive-deductive reasoning".[35]

Diagnoses are sometimes made in retrospect, when the treatment confirms the putative diagnosis. Consider the example of a patient who begins a consultation by saying, "Oh, its my sinuses doctor, I always end up having antibiotics for them". *Definitively* establishing the diagnosis of sinusitis in general practice is virtually impossible. The doctor may decide to offer antibiotics, but the reasons are not purely "evidence based": bacteriological studies may be impractical and unreliable; delaying treatment may cause an unnecessary prolongation of the pain or may cause the patient to loose money through absence from work. The doctor may also feel considerable pressure from the patient's expectations. Quite simply, the doctor's decision to prescribe antibiotics results from a balance of probabilities. But if the doctor prescribes antibiotics and the pain gets better, the diagnosis of sinusitis may be supported but is scarcely confirmed. Many illnesses are self limiting and are resolved by the body's own defences.

Non-diagnosis and non-disease

Bradley and Field argue that because it excludes "the undiagnosed" the application of EBM might be more limited in general practice than in specialist medicine.[15] The concept of non-disease is often encountered in general practice.[36 37] Indeed the problem of non-disease was dealt with in work widely held to be the "precursor" to the current EBM "movement". Non-disease exists when a specific disease is suspected on the basis of symptoms and signs but the investigation quite fails to confirm the original hypothesis.

GPs often use diagnostic labels that are less than descriptions of causes or understood pathologies. "It's just a virus" is often a shorthand way of referring to a condition whose fever and other symptoms are relatively mild, which is not life threatening, is self limiting, and does not require antibiotics. "Colic" and "abdominal migraine" are, similarly, descriptions of abdominal pains which are also self limiting and non-threatening but whose causes and processes remain obscure.

These labels should not be regarded as irresponsible or meaningless, rather, they represent a way of expressing an evolving, imprecise situation whose management is often best described as watchful waiting. These conditions may not be fully described in scientific terms, but the management of their uncertainties is as scientific as the present state of knowledge allows.

The relative infrequency of a fully realised "pathological" diagnosis in general practice is well documented. For example, in one study of nearly 4000 patients who presented in one year no firm diagnosis was made in 43% of cases.[38] Thomas coined the concept of the temporarily dependent patient—one which is poorly accommodated by EBM. In another study of 272 patients who presented to the GP with headaches only one third received a "diagnosis" after one year.[39]

Dealing with the areas of non-disease and non-diagnosis is a routine part of the GP's work. Some patients come to their doctor simply because they are "not feeling quite right".[40] This sense of unease may well herald the onset of a discreet illness but may also be the consequence of other forms of distress including unhappiness, tiredness, or unfavourable socioeconomic circumstances: "All aspects of human existence are the legitimate concerns of the general practitioner, provided they are presented as a problem by the patient".[41]

Others have argued that most interactions in general practice focus on issues which cannot be classified biomedically, except, perhaps, as "functional". One estimate suggests that two thirds of patients who consult in general practice do not have serious discreet pathology.[42] This does not diminish the legitimacy of their consultations, but it does signify that patients' perceptions have to be explored in a different way from that encompassed by the biomechanical model alone.

The danger in all this is that the very successes of EBM, where its application is most appropriate, could confuse us by suggesting that all clinical problem solving is synonymous with EBM. But it is not designed to deal with the problems of non-disease or the temporarily dependent patient. It is precisely in these very common clinical settings that the limitations of EBM in general practice become most evident.

The evidence in Evidence Based Medicine

EBM encourages the critical appraisal of the best available evidence to solve clinical problems.[43] For the most part, the evidence referred to is found in the results of randomised controlled trials or is collated in systematic reviews or meta-analyses. EBM has been criticised for relying too heavily on RCT,[44] and there have been serious reservations expressed about the methodology and validity of meta-analysis.[11 45]

The proponents of EBM are quite explicit about the importance of randomised controlled trials. It is argued that the breadth and explanatory power of a randomised controlled trial is the cornerstone not only for EBM but for evidence based public health, evidence based hospital administration, evidence based purchasing, and evidence based consumerism.[46]

In a randomised controlled trial a group of individuals (the study cohort) is identified by virtue of its members sharing a common characteristic—for example, a particular disease or risk factor. The researchers randomly allocate each member of the cohort to one or more study groups, each of which receives different interventions, preferably in a way that is not known to either the researcher or subject—so called "blinded intervention". After a period of time the outcome for each group is ascertained and the findings compared. Thus, RCT aggregate the benefits and disadvantages of alternative interventions in comparable populations within the same experimental environment.

The contribution of this type of clinical experiment has been huge, and the RCT has properly become the cornerstone of medical research. Large single trials have clarified the benefits of simple interventions: in one trial (ISIS-2) half of 17 000 patients enrolled benefited from taking low dose aspirin after they had had a heart attack compared with the group who were not given this treatment,[47] with the result that worldwide treatment patterns for this condition changed.[48]

Ellis *et al*[7] and Gill *et al*[9] cite evidence from RCT to support the treatment of conditions which are commonly encountered in both secondary and primary care—for example, unstable angina, congestive cardiac failure, asthma, eczema, and depression. And to help to appraise the strength of evidence critically from a particular RCT, the literature from the EBM Working Group provides useful guidance, clarifying in particular the clinical significance of outcome statistics.[46]

Yet numerous studies have documented the failure of doctors to apply new evidence from good clinical trials.[49,50] If the RCT is such a powerful technique, why this relative failure to incorporate its findings in general practice? The answer lies in the difficulties the GP faces in applying the evidence from RCT or megatrials. A first difficulty concerns the presentation, interpretation, and application of the outcome statistics from such trials. People who agree to enter a medical trial and sign a consent form may by that very act be expressing a particular, distinguishing characteristic which could prejudice the "representatives" of the trial population. Since the introduction of informed consent, which shifted enrolment decisions away from doctors to patients, the composition of populations in clinical trials has changed.[49,51]

In a clinical trial, a group of patients who share the same diagnosis may exhibit quite different patterns of illness behaviour; they may exhibit different symptoms or experience different severity or rates of progress of the subject condition. In randomised controlled trials, these individual experiences are grouped together for the sake of simplicity and clarity; the results are summated results from the combined experiences of a heterogeneous population of individual people.

Although the intention is to distribute potential biases equally between the two groups this does not eliminate the biases, it just disperses them. In this sense comparisons between the groups will be unbiased but run the risk of conflating several causal processes.[13]

A second difficulty concerns the relevance of the data from the population in the trial to the situation of the individual patient in the consulting room. To find out how far the results of a trial should apply to a particular patient the doctor has to know what kind of patients were in the trial, and the process of identifying the entry and exclusion criteria in a trial can take a lot of time and effort. Although the EBM Working Group do offer guidelines to explain this process,[52] the authors selected as an explanatory model the results of a trial which have been criticised elsewhere for excluding over 93% of the initially eligible group of patients—over 1000 on unspecified administrational grounds.[53 54]

Most clinical trials are quite narrow in their scope and carefully select their population for maximum responsiveness to the intervention.[49] In everyday clinical practice the strict application of the entry criteria to a RCT can exclude patients from the benefits of treatment. Haynes offers the example of two patients admitted to his clinical service with cardiac problems. The first, a 78 year old woman, had breathlessness, was found to be in heart failure, but did not have any chest pain. The second, a 50 year old man, had severe chest pain (suggesting a heart attack) but his electrocardiogram did not show significant changes. Neither received streptokinase (a drug given to disperse the blood clot causing the problem) because neither patient presented with the very strict eligibility criteria of the definitive studies that had demonstrated the medicine's benefits. Subsequently, both patients were in fact found by further tests to have suffered heart attacks.[49]

The problem for all clinicians in using the results of EBM is simply this. Faced with a patient's particular clinical problem the doctor needs to know if the outcome statistic from a relevant trial will apply to *this* patient, in *this* consultation, in *this* particular environment. These vital questions, however, are unanswerable. Outcome statistics reflect the *average* experience of each group; extrapolating from that group average to a single patient's chances is impossible. What can be judged is the average order of probability in a large group of people whose personal and disease characteristics bear a resemblance to those of the patient. What cannot be estimated is the actual patient specific risk.

The analogy can be drawn with a diversified financial portfolio. A balanced financial portfolio is a good idea because aggregate outcome is what matters—there will be winners and losers within the portfolio over a period of time. As long as, overall, there are more winners than losers the idea is acceptable. But such aggregation does not make sense if one is concerned about each individual constituent of the portfolio. This is what happens when one tries to apply the evidence from a population to an individual.

In a randomised controlled trial the individuals may have had varying experiences which, when summated, will produce the outcome statistic for the RCT. Even if the outcome statistic describes a benefit for the intervention the practitioner is left with the possibility that the intervention may produce a negative outcome in the particular individual. And although the trial outcome may be "statistically significant" (that is, not attributable to chance), the practitioner is left wondering if that also means that it is clinically significant (that is, relevant to the patient's unique problem). The common application by doctors of the term "significant" to both population statistics and the individual clinical picture can thus cause confusion. This is what Schon is talking about when he compares the "hard, high ground" of research based theory to the "swampy lowlands where situations are confusing messes".[55]

While "statistically significant" results of relevant trials can help the doctor to assess the *order* of risks to the patient, what is the patient to make of such figures? What is the woman with breast cancer to make of the "statistical" statement that 34 women with the disease have to be treated with tamoxifen to save one life?[56] In addition to considering statistical and clinical significance the need for a third sort of significance in the problem solving dialogue becomes evident. This could be termed personal significance. It may be unwise to assume that what is statistically significant to the researcher and clinically significant to the doctor will also be personally significant to the patient.

Consider the rationale for treating hypertension in a middle aged man. One could explain to such a patient that 170 middle aged men would have to have their blood pressure treated for five years to prevent one stroke. The patient may well elect to take his chances with the other 169 rather than accept the sick role of a patient requiring daily medication for the rest of his life.

People's attitudes to health are not necessarily or exclusively logical. A person's attitude to health and the actions taken on that basis are determined by how the person perceives a particular threat to health, the strength of belief in the advantages of changing behaviour to accommodate that threat, and how difficult the patient believes that behavioural change will be. The beliefs that form attitudes to health are influenced by personal, family, social, and demographic factors.[57] An individual's actions based on these personal health beliefs are not always apparently rational.[58] For example, research has demonstrated a correlation between the frequency of prescribing psychotropic drugs for mothers and the frequency of prescribing antibiotics for their children on account of respiratory infections.[59] People are influenced in the actions they take by what they think others might expect them to do and by how much importance they attach to that.[60] Doctors are people too; they are not immunised by their medical education from the cultural, societal, and psychological influences which form attitudes to health.

Systematic reviews and meta-analysis

Systematic reviews, which include meta-analyses, were developed in response to the huge quantity of information which was becoming available in print. The rationale for systematic review is based on the following five points:[61]

- Systematic reviews separate unsound information from more worthy studies and can be used by clinicians to keep abreast of the literature
- There is evidence that continuously updating the literature through systematic review shortens the time interval between initial publication of new clinical material and its proper implementation into clinical practice; the Oxford database of perinatal trials is one example of this[62]
- Systematic reviews can help by evaluating the extent to which the information from clinical studies is generalisable; here systematic reviews have an interpretative function, recognising the diversity of sources from individual studies
- They can also evaluate the consistency, or otherwise, of relations between individual studies
- Systematic reviews whose methodology is explicitly described can assess more accurately the state of knowledge in a particular clinical specialty.

Meta-analyses, which provide such systematic overview, pool the findings of comparable studies to obtain an overall picture. Such overviews, it is argued, minimise random errors in the evaluation of treatments because more patients are involved in the overview than in any single trial.[63] The technique of meta-analysis was developed partly because of the problems of generalisation from randomised controlled trials and partly because the sheer volume of

RCT was becoming unmanageable. Developments in information technology now permit systematic reviews, which can be lengthy documents when printed, to be published electronically.[59]

Guidelines for assessing the strengths and weaknesses of meta-analyses have been proposed.[64,65] Advocates assert that it is a statistically objective and explicit technique and describe the following key principles:

- Firstly, a meta-analysis should be comprehensive and include all trials concerning the subject condition not just those which are published
- Secondly, a meta-analysis should include all data on an intention to treat basis; this means that all the patients in a particular trial allocated to one treatment (even if for some subsequent reason they did not actually receive it) should be compared at the end with all the patients in the other group
- Thirdly, a meta-analysis should obtain information on all subgroups and data on complete follow up. This last criterion acknowledges the fact that the results of RCT can become frozen in time, and a meta-analysis, written at a later date, might offer a further overview of a particular group of patients whose outcome may modify the reported trial effect
- Finally, meta-analyses should calculate their statistics derived from data on individual patients rather than aggregate data.

The strength of the methodology of a meta-analysis is crucial, and ideally all the steps in the process, from the literature search, through the criteria for including studies, and any calculations used should be explicitly stated. Good meta-analyses can properly and substantially influence treatment strategies. One example of a meta-analysis that has influenced clinical practice is the overview of trials of adjuvant therapy in early breast cancer.[66] Taken separately, none of the trials on early breast cancer had been large enough to provide reliable evidence on long term survival. Taken together, a clearer difference in 10 year survival rates between the study and the control populations emerged.[48] Another landmark meta-analysis demonstrated the effectiveness of intravenous streptokinase in the treatment of heart attacks.[67]

Concerns have been expressed that meta-analysis may not be an exact statistical science.[12] Firstly, even after painstaking detective work has uncovered all the published and unpublished studies on a topic the problem of heterogeneity between the grouped studies remains. Secondly, a consensus on what to include in a meta-analysis can be difficult to achieve. There is a large variety of study designs, types of treatment evaluations, categories of patients involved, and calculation of outcomes. Here, the analytical process in meta-analysis can become less statistically explicit and more interpretative and subjective. The ways in which studies for inclusion in a meta-analysis are weighted has been described as too arbitrary.[12] Here again there may be an element of interpretation: which should be down weighted more, trials with poor blinding or trials with incomplete follow up?

Also, meta-analyses have at times provided misleading information. The example which the *Drugs and Therapeutic Bulletin*[68] used to explain the basis of the technique dealt with an intervention—the effects of intravenous magnesium on mortality in patients with suspected myocardial infarction—which subsequent mega-trials showed to be ineffective.[69] In 1988 misleading meta-analyses also suggested that routine use of nitrate might be beneficial in treating myocardial infarctions. But subsequent trials (ISIS 4, GISSI 3) directly researched the question and found only non-significant differences between the intervention and the control groups. This has led to the suggestion that meta-analysis is better regarded as a tool for generating hypotheses rather than for testing them.[65]

To summarise, meta-analysis is a technique that provides a more precise quantitative estimate of an effect that is already known to exist from the RCTs that are combined to construct the analysis. It is not a way of defining causation in medicine but can permit general qualitative conclusions to be drawn about a class of drugs or a treatment.[13] Meta-analyses cannot tell clinicians how to treat individual patients; the results of such analyses are even more difficult to apply to individuals than the RCT that are combined to produce them.

Systematic reviews of evidence from research will continue to play an increasing part in the evolution of health services and in the justification of funding. They will also contribute to the education of non-medical health care professionals and lay people. From the point of view of general practice, however, their limitations must always be considered alongside their evident benefits.

Measuring the measurable

The description of EBM[4] and the illustration of its application were criticised[7] for posing only questions the answers to which could be measured and therefore for implying that if something can not be measured it is of little value. Are these criticisms justified?

Certainly in medical practice there is an obligation to measure, as accurately as one can, the strength of an observation, a diagnostic test, or a management decision. The EBM Working Group set themselves to these tasks and published helpful articles on all three of these topics.[52 70 71]

If a diagnosis or treatment is to be determined by a quantitative observation it is critically important that it is based on the best available evidence. Consider the following example, taken from one of the articles in the users' guide series, published in the *Journal of the American Medical Association* by the EBM Working Group.[72]

> Mrs J is a 76 year old retired school teacher who consults because she thinks she is becoming forgetful. The doctor's assessment includes a formal test of her mental state and a series of biochemical tests, the results of which are all normal; this confirms that the patient is suffering from dementia. Her son asks to see the doctor about the problem.

The authors of the article suggest the kind of questions which the son might ask the doctor in this situation, questions which can be appropriately dealt with by EBM. They explore two questions: What is my mother's prognosis? and Will my mother be alive in five years? They then go on to show how a rigorous appraisal of the relevant literature can produce quantifiable answers to these two questions.

The selection of these questions is instructive because they can provide answers that are expressed numerically. Yet patients, or their representatives, also pose different types of questions, some of which have numerate answers, but others that are more reflective, philosophical, or existential.[41] The problem of the nature of research questions is touched on in a trenchant critique of academic research in clinical medicine, which argues that the requirements of medical research are limited by insisting "that an answer should be numeric, otherwise it is not a real answer".[73]

Consider again the example of the 76 year old woman with dementia. The patient's son may ask the general practitioner, Can my mother be cured, will she die, can her suffering be relieved? The answers to these questions will certainly involve skills set out usefully by the EBM Working Group. But he may also ask, Why has this happened to her? and What will happen to us now? He may well reflect on the impact that the mother's illness will have on his own family: Should mother come and stay with us? What will the effect be on my marriage if she does?

It is not always possible to formulate from the patient's presenting story a question the answer to which is available from biomedical research. This difference is not to be interpreted as an inherent weakness of EBM: the science of EBM does not exclude humanity. But it illustrates that it is not constructed to deal with the broader qualitative issues of clinical problem solving or to provide the skill to deal supportively with them.

From the point of view of general practice the anxiety is that an overemphasis on the questions that can be asked and answered by EBM may run the risk of devaluing those questions that cannot be so expressed.[15] The consultation in general practice is not simply a place where a patient seeks scientific answers to questions. Toon states: "The consultation is the patient's forum for coming to understand her illness, not merely a rational understanding, but an understanding which involves the emotions and which contributes to the growth of the individual".[74] In a patient centred consultation, the doctor recognises this and tries to see the illness through the patient's eyes.[75] Patients' questions are answered partly by reference to science but also to what Heath calls "the search for meaning".[41]

The nature of general practice

Any experience that an individual perceives as threatening or problematic and introduces to the consultation becomes the legitimate concern of the general practitioner. Being competent to deal with the range of potential problems in general practice requires a portfolio of intellectual, professional, and personal skills. Some aspects of the general practitioner's competence have been described as doctor centred.[76] They include curative and rehabilitative care, promoting health, and organising preventive activities. Personal skills are equally important components of competence but until recently have received less attention. They are the more patient centred qualities of competence and include moral and personal attributes.

In the United States, the American Board of Internal Medicine stated that "A major responsibility of training residents in internal medicine is to stress the importance of the humanistic qualities in the relationship between the patient and physician".[77] In the United Kingdom it is recommended that "the recertification of all clinicians should include an assessment of honesty, self-awareness in the professional context, empathy, respect for patient autonomy and confidentiality".[78]

An important ingredient of general practice is the formation of a human relationship between the doctor and the patient. Forming such a relationship is the basis for good consulting, and it requires the ability to identify imaginatively with what a patient experiences subjectively during an illness and recognising the validity and importance of that experience for the patient.[41 73] The term "human relationship" is used here with a specific meaning to distinguish it from the term "personal relationship".

For doctors this distinction is important. In a *personal relationship* two human beings decide spontaneously to exchange benign sentiments based on mutual care, concern, and affection. As the relationship develops, the mutuality and reciprocity grow more profound on both sides; the way in which a personal relationship develops depends on the equal participation of both parties. In a *human relationship* one person, responding to the human condition of another, seeks to initiate an exchange of benign sentiments.[79] Human relationships require a genuine concern from the instigator and a positive response from the participant. Such relationships are based on self knowledge, tolerance, self confidence, patience, and the ability to listen and communicate.

In human relationships the depth of feelings and personal involvement should never be as profound as in a personal relationship; for doctors there is a duty to maintain these relationships at the appropriate level. It is this element of control, maintaining the relationship at the appropriate level, which epitomises the difference between the two types of relationship. To illustrate how the tasks of applying best evidence and forming human relationships can be combined, consider this example.

> Bert, a former professional soldier, is 63 years old. He consults one day saying he feels low. The doctor carries out a standard depression inventory to confirm the diagnosis based on Bert's symptoms and identifies Bert as a "case" of depression. Calling on the evidence from clinical trials he prescribes a tricyclic antidepressant.

Here, the appropriate use of EBM helps the doctor arrive at the diagnosis of "depression" by using a validated instrument and helps the patient to benefit from the best treatment suggested by the relevant clinical trials. Speaking further to Bert, the doctor establishes that the depression was initiated by his son's failure to get into the army. Bert had been a soldier himself, loved the army, and had always wanted his son to join the same regiment. His son also wanted to do this, but when the son failed he became antisocial, drinking too much, and experimenting with soft drugs. Bert had found the experience devastating.

This example illustrates the three levels at which a doctor can understand and empathise with a patient. At the first level, the doctor categorises the patient on the basis of established, recognisable patterns of disease: Bert is a "case" of depression. At the second level, the doctor makes use of the patient's life history to try to understand what has been happening to him: Bert's aspirations for his son are based on his own experiences as a soldier. At the third level, the doctor recognises the uniqueness of the patient's human condition and the *significance* and gravity of the illness from the patient's perspective.

Accordingly, in this consultation the use of EBM and the formation of the human relationship are both necessary ingredients of a productive consultation. Neither the diagnostic technique nor the relationship building skills are in themselves sufficient to constitute a good consultation. Heath identifies two fundamental roles for the general practitioner. These are acting as interpreter and guardian at the interface between illness and disease and acting as a witness to the patient's experience of both.[41]

Consider the patient with end stage chronic obstructive airways disease, for whom no more can be done by the respiratory specialists. Such patients may linger for months or years in a terminal state, deriving gradually diminishing benefit from steroids, antibiotics, and bronchodilators. Their burden of illness and that on their carers has to be witnessed and supported despite the failure of biomedicine to help them.

General practitioners have to distinguish between illness and disease; illness may exist without disease, which is a narrower reconfiguration of the patient's story based on biomedical science.[26] Doctors have a duty to explore the meaning of illness, recognising its potential origin in unhappiness, unfavourable socioeconomic factors, or in chronically unsatisfactory personal relationships. They have to recognise that the severity of an illness can be a function of an individual's health beliefs and particular life circumstances.[57]

There is a further duty to protect patients from overenthusiastic interpretation of illness as disease; Kleinman cautions doctors against the "over-literal interpretation of accounts best understood metaphorically". Here, the doctor works with the patient to make sense of the patient's experience in the context of the rest of the patient's life. This has been described elsewhere as the hermeneutic[74] or biographical[80] tasks of the doctor.

The place of Evidence Based Medicine in general practice

The EBM Working Group argues that many patients are being denied the benefits of evidence from well conducted clinical trials.[43] The evidence supports this.[50] Accordingly, there is a responsibility for doctors to acquire new skills in accessing, evaluating, and applying the results of the vast number of clinical studies now being published worldwide. In pursuit of this end, the integration of EBM into the clinical work of general practice is both necessary and timely.

The risk lies in regarding EBM as the only and last word in the pursuit of clinical quality and the search for relevant evidence. For example, the conventional approach to the task of modifying the behaviour of doctors has been to offer educational inputs or formulate clinical guidelines. To some extent these work.[81] But the decision to change a clinical habit can be the result of a series of influences, which may not be dealt with by a conventional approach where the researcher has to guess in advance which intervention is most likely to succeed.

A recent study of doctors' reasons for changing their prescribing behaviour illustrates this point.[82] The researchers encouraged the clinicians to explain and understand their own reasons for altering their prescribing habits. The researchers identified three models of change. Some doctors altered their prescribing policy as a result of the sheer weight of pressure to move in a certain direction, evidence for which came in various forms, such as articles, letters from consultants, or talks that they attended. A second model of change was more abrupt and came in response to near "clinical disasters" or in response to changes in prescribing initiated by a second doctor, sometimes a locum. A third group of doctors seemed to embrace change in general more enthusiastically. They were more prepared to be influenced by a variety of sources, some of which would be regarded as conventionally authoritative, like journal articles, but others were not, like magazine adverts or television programmes.

What this important paper suggests is obvious but profound: that it is vital to define the nature of a problem before identifying the solution. EBM may help to make some diagnoses and treatments in general practice more safe but it cannot cover the full range of diagnostic and therapeutic issues that make up so much of the work of general practice. As EBM becomes more widely integrated into general practice this should not occur at the expense of encouraging the search for other approaches to changing clinical behaviour.[58 83] GPs express two further anxieties about EBM. The first concerns the medicolegal implications of the publication of rigorous systematic reviews and consequent guidelines. The second concerns the managerial implications of the widespread adoption of EBM in general practice.

Will failure to adhere to a highly authoritative systematic review or a published clinical guideline be deemed negligent? This question is all the more pertinent in the light of the recent award of £825 000 against the doctor who advised the mother of a child who had had convulsions not to have the child immunised—with disastrous consequences for the child.[84] The present position is that a witness in a legal case may refer to written protocols or guidelines when citing evidence about accepted standards of care. Because written guidelines are classified as hearsay evidence (and so cannot be cross examined), however, a judge cannot decide what is "reasonable care" simply by referring to them.[85]

Increasingly, doctors recognise the importance of respecting the patient's autonomy and are appropriately encouraging patients to participate more actively in decisions that affect their health. This may lead to circumstances in which the patient disagrees with a doctor's preferred (evidence based) option. What is to be the touchstone of "reasonable care"—the product of EBM or the product of the doctor's negotiation with the patient?

Consider the example of an elderly woman who has hypertension and is discovered to be in atrial fibrillation. The doctor considers the accumulated evidence on the management of atrial fibrillation and decides that anticoagulation with warfarin is the preferred option.[86] The elderly woman, however, lives alone, finds it very difficult to come to the surgery for blood tests, and does not have a telephone. She does not want to pester her neighbours by asking them to telephone in for her blood test results. She decides against taking warfarin. How is the doctor to respond? How much pressure should the doctor put on this patient to agree to the medical strategy supported by powerful evidence from RCT?

The results of the same RCT on the use of warfarin in atrial fibrillation have come to the attention of senior managers in the NHS. They have identified anticoagulant treatment for patients with atrial fibrillation as a key element in purchasing negotiations for health authority corporate contracts.[87] Here, the managers can be seen as responding to good scientific evidence. But their translation of good research evidence into the terms of a contract is inappropriate if it fails to take account of human variation.[54] If insensitively interpreted, the management implications of EBM could leave doctors (and their patients) between a rock and a hard place.

Two examples of the application of EBM referred to widely in this chapter also have management implications. These retrospective audits of decision making in clinical practice have suggested that about 80% of the decisions were evidence based.[7 9] Does this become the benchmark against which other practices will be judged? Will health authorities require a minimum acceptable level of evidence based decisions by GPs and hospital doctors? And how will they make such judgments?

Both EBM and a sensitive understanding of the patient's unique predicament are prerequisites of good general practice—but at present only the former can be measured. While this does not invalidate the task of forming human relationships, there remain concerns that transactions which cannot be measured may be regarded as less valuable than those that can.[15] Mary Midgeley states: "The mere presence of an emotional factor in any kind of decision does not take it out of the realm of rational thought. All our thinking involves emotional factors as well as rational ones, just as every physical object has size as well as shape. These are not alternatives. The presence of one does not mean the absence of another".[89]

EBM presents three challenges for general practice. Firstly, those concerned in the education and training of GPs have a responsibility to make available workshops on EBM which convey the advantages of the method *in the unique context of general practice.* But the advent of EBM increases the responsibility to teach GPs about the metaphysical aspects of the consultation: the importance of using humility and compassion, of witnessing and empathising with a fellow human being's suffering.

Secondly, those who are responsible for funding research should support well designed projects which seek to explain and change clinicians' behaviour in ways which acknowledge *the particular nature and context* of the problems those clinicians encounter.

Thirdly, the practising doctor is now challenged to integrate EBM into the strong humanitarian tradition of general practice. Midgeley covers this need thus: "We need ways of thinking which are unifying enough to give us guiding patterns, but not so strongly reductive as to leave out something important".[89]

In her article outlining the rationale for systematic reviews, Mulrow quotes TS Eliot from *The Rock*: "Where is the knowledge we have lost in information". For general practice a fuller quotation from this section of *The Rock* illustrates better the challenge of evidence in clinical medicine:

> "Where is the life we have lost in living,
> Where is the wisdom we have lost in knowledge,
> Where is the knowledge we have lost in information?"

1 Evidence Based Medicine Working Group. Evidence based medicine: a new approach to teaching the practice of medicine. *JAMA* 1992;**268**:2420–5.
2 Oxman AD, Sackett D, Guyatt GH. Users' guide to the medical literature. I. How to get started. *JAMA* 1993;**270**:2093–5.
3 Davidoff F, Haynes B, Sackett D, *et al.* Evidence based medicine (editorial). *BMJ* 1995;**310**:1085–6.
4 Rosenberg W, Donald A. Evidence based medicine: an approach to clinical problem solving. *BMJ* 1995;**310**:1122–6.
5 Sackett DL, Rosenberg WMC, Muir Gray JA, *et al.* Evidence based medicine: what it is and what it isn't. *BMJ* 1996;**312**:71–2.
6 Dawes MG. On the need for evidence based general and family practice. *Evidence Based Medicine* 1996;**1**:68–9.
7 Ellis J, Mulligan I, Rowe J, *et al.* In-patient general medicine is evidence based. *Lancet* 1995;**346**:407–10.
8 Guyatt GH, Rennie D. Users' guide to the medical literature. *JAMA* 1993; **270**:2096–7.
9 Gill P, Dowell AC, Neal RD, *et al.* Evidence based general practice: a retrospective study of interventions in one training practice. *BMJ* 1996;**312**: 819–21.
10 Iggo N. Evidence based medicine (letter). *Lancet* 1995;**346**:839.
11 Charlton BG. Megatrials are subordinate to medical science (letter). *BMJ* 1995; **311**:257.
12 Thompson SG, Pocock SJ. Can meta-analysis be trusted? *Lancet* 1991;**338**: 1127–30.
13 Carlton BG. The uses and abuses of meta-analysis. *Fam Med* (in press).

14 Fowler PBS. Evidence based medicine (letter). *Lancet* 1995;**346**:838.
15 Bradley F, Field J. Evidence based medicine (letter). *Lancet* 1995;**346**:838–9.
16 Smith BH. Quality cannot always be quantified (letter). *BMJ* 1995;**311**:258.
17 Kuhn TS. *The structure of scientific revolutions.* Chicago: University of Chicago Press, 1970.
18 McWhinney IR. Changing models: the impact of Kuhn's theory on medical practice. *Fam Pract* 1983;**1**:3–8.
19 Sackett DL, Haines RB, Tugwell P. *Clinical epidemiology.* Boston: Little, Brown, 1985.
20 Lilienfield AM, Lilienfield DE. A century of case controlled studies: progress? *Journal of Chronic Diseases* 1979;**32**:5–13.
21 Cochrane AL. *Effectiveness and efficiency: random reflections on health services.* London: Nuffield Provincial Hospital Trust, 1971. (Rock Carling Fellowship.)
22 Armenian HK, Lilienfield DE. Overview and historical perspective. *Epidemiol Rev* 1994;**16**:1–5.
23 Lilienfield DE, Stolley PD. *Foundations of epidemiology.* 3rd ed. New York: Oxford University Press, 1994.
24 Doll R, Hill AB. Smoking and carcinoma of the lung: preliminary report. *BMJ* 1950;ii:1225–36.
25 Silagy C, Jewell D. Review of 39 years of randomised controlled trials in the British Journal of General Practice. *Br J Gen Pract* 1994;**44**:359–63.
26 Kleinman A. *The illness narrative.* New York: Basic Books, 1988.
27 Balint M. *The doctor, his patient, and the illness.* New York: International Universities Press, 1957.
28 Elstein AS, Kagan N, Hulman D, *et al.* Methods and theory in the study of medical enquiry. *Journal of Medical Education* 1972;**47**:87–92.
29 Howie JGR. Diagnosis: the Achilles' heel? *J R Coll Gen Pract* 1972;**22**:310–5.
30 Marinker M. Balint seminars and vocational training in general practice. *J R Coll Gen Pract* 1970;**19**:79.
31 Williamson JW, Goldschmidt PG, Jilson IA. *Information demonstration project: final report.* Baltimore: Policy Research, 1979.
32 Royal College of General Practitioners. *The future general practitioner. Learning and teaching.* London: RCGP, 1972.
33 Marinker M. Clinical method. In: Cormack J, Marinker M, Morrell D, eds. *Teaching clinical method.* London: Kluwer Medical, 1981.
34 McWhinney IR. Problem solving and decision making. In: *An introduction to family medicine.* Oxford: Oxford University Press, 80–105.
35 Willis J. *The paradox of progress.* Oxford: Radcliffe Medical Press, 1995.
36 Scott AJ. Diagnostic accuracy would be improved by developing more categories of non-disease. *Medical Hypotheses* 1977;**3**:135–7.
37 Dixon AS. There is a lot of it about: clinical strategies in family practice. *J R Coll Gen Pract* 1986;**36**:468–71.
38 Thomas KB. Temporarily dependent patients in general practice. *BMJ* 1974; i:59–65.
39 Bass MJ, Dempsey B, McWhinney IR. The natural history of headaches in family practice. In: Proceedings of the 10th World Conference of the World Organisation of National Colleges and Academies of General Practitioners, Singapore, 1983.
40 Rudebeck CE. General practice and the dialogue of clinical practice: on symptoms, symptom presentation and bodily empathy. *Scan J Prim Health Care* 1992;suppl 1.
41 Heath I. *The mystery of general practice.* London: Nuffield Provincial Hospitals Trust, 1995.
42 Kellner R. Functional somatic symptoms and hypochondriasis. *Arch Gen Psych* 1985;**42**:821–33.

43 Sackett DL, Rosenburg WCM. The need for evidence based medicine. *J R Soc Med* 1995;**88**:620–4.
44 Charlton BG. Medical practice and the double blind randomised controlled trial. *Br J Gen Pract* 1992;**42**:355–6.
45 Charlton BG. Practice guidelines and practical judgment: the role of mega-trials, meta-analysis and consensus. *Br J Gen Pract* 1994;**44**:290–1.
46 Sackett DL, Cook RJ. Understanding clinical trials (editorial). *BMJ* 1994;**309**: 755–6.
47 ISIS-2 (Second International Study of Infarct Survival Collaborative Group). Randomised trial of intravenous streptokinase, oral aspirin, both, or neither among 17,187 cases of suspected acute myocardial infarction. *Lancet* 1988;ii: 349–60.
48 Collins R, Peto R, Gray R, *et al.* In: Weatherall DJ, Ledingham JGG, Warrell DA, eds. *The Oxford textbook of medicine.* Oxford: Oxford University Press, 1996:21–32.
49 Haynes RB. Some problems in applying clinical evidence. In: Warren KS, Mosteller F, eds. *Doing more good than harm: the evaluation of health care interventions.* New York: Annals of New York Academy of Science, 1993: 210–24.
50 Haines A, Jones R. Implementing findings in research. *BMJ* 1994;**308**:1488–92.
51 Silverman WA, Altamn DG. Patients' preferences and randomised trials. *Lancet* 1996;**347**:171–4.
52 Guyatt GH, Sackett DL, Cook DJ. Users' guide the medical literature. II. How to use an article about therapy or prevention. *JAMA* 1994;**271**:59–63.
53 Ezekowtiz MD, Bridgers SL, James KE, *et al*, for the Veterans Affairs/Prevention in Non-rheumatic Atrial Fibrillation Investigators. Warfarin in the prevention of stroke associated with non-rheumatic atrial fibrillation. *N Engl J Med* 1992; **327**:1406–12.
54 Sweeney KG, Pereira Gray DJ, Steele RJF, *et al.* The use of warfarin in non-rheumatic atrial fibrillation: a commentary from general practice. *Br J Gen Pract* 1995;**45**:253–8.
55 Schon DA. *The reflective practitioner: how professionals think in action.* 3rd ed. Kings Lynn: Basic Books, 1995.
56 Feinstein A. Meta-analysis: statistical alchemy for the 21st century. *J Clin Epidemiol* 1995;**48**:71–9.
57 Becker MH. The health belief model and sick role of behaviour. *Health Education Monographs* 1974;**2**:409–19.
58 Johnston M. Health related behaviour change. In: *Preventing coronary heart disease in primary care.* London: Kings Fund, 1995:37,47.
59 Howie JGR, Bigg AR. Family trends in psychotropic and antibiotic prescribing in general practice. *BMJ* 1980;**280**:86-8.3.
60 Fishbein M, Azjen I. *Belief, attitude, intention and behavior.* New York: Wiley, 1975.
61 Mulrow CD. Rationale for systematic reviews. *BMJ* 1994;**309**:597–9.
62 Chalmers I, Hetherington J, Newdick M, *et al.* The Oxford database of perinatal trials: developing a register of published reports of controlled trials. *Control Clin Trials* 1986;**7**:306–24.
63 West RR. A look at the statistical overview (or meta-analysis). *J R Coll Physicians Lond* 1993;**27**:111–5.
64 Egger M, Davey Smith G. Misleading meta-analysis. *BMJ* 1995;**310**:752–4.
65 Borzak S, Ridler PM. Discordance between meta-analysis and large scale randomised controlled trials. *Ann Intern Med* 1995;**123**:873–7.
66 Early Breast Cancer Trialists' Collaborative Group. Systematic treatment of early breast cancer by hormonal, cytotoxic or immune therapy: 133 randomised

trials, involving 31,000 recurrences and 24,000 deaths among 75,000 women. *Lancet* 1992;**339**:1–15,71–85.

67 Fibrinolytic Therapy Trialists' Group. Indications for fibrinolytic therapy in suspected myocardial infarction: collaborative overview of early mortality and major morbidity results from all randomised trials over 1000 patients. *Lancet* 1994;**343**:311–22.

68 Anon. Systematical overview of controlled trials (meta-analysis) help us to clarify treatment effects. *Drug Ther Bull* 1992;**30**:March 7.

69 Teo KK, Yusuf S, Colling R, *et al.* Effects of intravenous magnesium in suspected acute myocardial infarction: overview of randomised trials. *BMJ* 1991;**303**: 1499–503.

70 Sackett DL. A primer on the precision and accuracy of the clinical examination. *JAMA* 1992;**267**:2638–44.

71 Jaeschke R, Guyatt G, Sackett DL, for the Evidence Based Medicine Working Group. How to use an article about a diagnostic test. *JAMA* 1994;**271**:389–91.

72 Laupacis A, Wells G, Scott Richardson W, *et al.* How to use an article about prognosis. *JAMA* 1994;**272**:234–7.

73 Rudebeck CE. Humanism in medicine: benevolence or realism? *Scand J Prim Health Care* 1992;**10**:161–2.

74 Toon P. *What is good general practice?* Exeter: Royal College of General Practitioners, 1994. (Occasional paper No 65.)

75 Peppiat R. Eliciting parents' views of the cause of their problems: a practical strategy for general practitioners. *Fam Pract* 1992;**9**:295–8.

76 Guilbert JJ. Educational objectives. In: *Educational handbook for health care personnel.* Geneva: WHO, 1987. (No 35.)

77 American Board of Internal Medicine. Subcommittee of the evaluation of humanistic qualities in the internist. *A guide to awareness and evaluation*: ABIM, Washington 1985.

78 Southgate L, Jolly B. Determining the content of recertification procedures. In: Newble D, Wakeford R, Jolly B, eds. *The certification and recertification of doctors.* Cambridge: Cambridge University Press, 1994.

79 Sweeney BJ. *Is there an expertise in human relationship?* Glasgow: University of Glasgow, 1992. (MPhil thesis.)

80 Marinker M. *The end of general practice.* London: Royal College of Physicians, 1994. (Bayliss lecture.)

81 Grimshaw JM, Russell IT. Effect of clinical guidelines on medical practice: a systematic review of rigorous evaluations. *Lancet* 1993;**342**:1317–22.

82 Armstrong D, Reyburn H, Jones R. A study of general practitioners' reasons for changing their prescribing behaviour. *BMJ* 1996;**312**:494–5.

83 Rollinick S, Kinnersly P, Stott N. Methods of helping patients with behaviour change. *BMJ* 1993;**307**:188–90.

84 Anon. Legal warning on £825k measles award against GP. *Pulse* 1996;April 13: 8.

85 Hurwitz B. Clinical guidelines and the law (editorial). *BMJ* 1996;**311**:1517–8.

86 Atrial Fibrillation Investigators. Risk factors for stroke and efficacy of antithrombitic treatment in atrial fibrillation: analysis of pooled data from randomised controlled trials. *Arch Intern Med* 1994;**154**:1449–57.

87 NHS Management Executive. *First steps for the NHS.* London: Department of Health, 1992.

88 Midgley M. *Science as salvation: a modern myth and its meaning.* London: Routledge, 1992.

The Partners:

Channel Four and University of York

The Question:

How can the mass communications media inform the public debate about health care policy?

The Writers:

Vicki Entwistle, Research Fellow, University of York
Ian S Watt, Dissemination Manager, University of York
Richard Bradbury, Research Assistant, University of York
Lesley J Pehl, Research Fellow, University of York

Think Tank Members:

(*The group met only once, after which it was decided to tackle the question by commissioning the research that is here presented.*)

Ms Karen Brown (Chair), Controller of Factual Programmes, Channel 4
Professor Julian Tudor Hart, Visiting Professor, Royal Free Hospital Medical School
Ms Sylvia Hines, Deputy Commissioning Editor in Education, Channel 4
Baroness Margaret Jay, Opposition Principal Spokesperson on Health
Professor Marshall Marinker, Visiting Professor of General Practice, UMDS, London and Advisor in Health Care Policy and Medical Education, MSD Ltd
Ms Becky Miles, Chair, National Cancer Alliance
Professor Richard Smith, Editor, British Medical Journal

Individuals Subsequently Consulted:

Sir Cyril Chantler, Dr Bruce Charlton, Ms Angela Coulter, Louise Dilner, Professor John Durant, Dr Jonathan Glover, Mr Philip Hunt, Mr Simon Jenkins, Mr Chris Longley, Professor Lewis Wolpert

5 The media and the message

How did the media cover the Child B case?

VIKKI A ENTWISTLE, IAN S WATT,
RICHARD BRADBURY, LESLEY J PEHL

The recent case of a girl with leukaemia, known for legal reasons as Child B, highlighted among other things the complex and difficult nature of decisions about the treatment of children diagnosed as being terminally ill. In the first part of this chapter we report on a study of media coverage of this case from March to December 1995, paying particular attention to the arguments presented in support of or against Child B receiving particular treatments and of those treatments being funded by the NHS. In the second part we discuss some of the issues raised by the media coverage of the case and by the case itself. The first two parts were written before it was announced in May 1996 that Child B had died. In the final part of the chapter, we describe and discuss how the media covered the death of Child B.

Outline of the Child B case

Child B recovered from non-Hodgkin's lymphoma and acute lymphoblastic leukaemia but subsequently developed acute myeloid leukaemia. In January 1995, when she was 10, her father was told by NHS consultants at both Addenbrookes and the Royal Marsden hospitals that she had about six to eight weeks to live. They said that the only possible treatment, intensive chemotherapy and a bone marrow transplant (which would be her second), was very unlikely to succeed and would have such distressing side effects that they could not recommend it as being in her best interests.

Child B's father did not accept this decision. He sought opinions from other doctors in the United Kingdom and America and found a consultant in London who was prepared to treat his daughter in the private sector. His local health authority, Cambridge, however, refused to grant an extra contractual referral to fund the treatment, which would have cost £75 000. (Cambridge Health Authority was part of Cambridge and Huntingdon Health Commission, whose officers handled the case and from whom press statements were issued. For simplicity's sake and in keeping with the dominant use in the media, we have used "the health authority" for both organisations.) The father challenged this refusal in court, at which point the pseudonym Child B was given to conceal the girl's identity and protect her from the knowledge of how ill she was. The High Court ruled on 10 March 1995 that the health authority should reconsider their decision, but Appeal Court judges later that day overturned the High Court ruling and said that the health authority had acted rationally and fairly in making their decision.

The case attracted much publicity, and an anonymous benefactor provided the money for the treatment her father wanted. Child B was given intensive chemotherapy privately by Dr Peter Gravett, who subsequently thought that this was not successful enough to warrant performing a second bone marrow transplant. Instead, he treated Child B with an unevaluated treatment called donor lymphocyte infusion.

The treatment was apparently successful in the short term. Child B went into remission and survived longer than most medical professionals had predicted she would. The health authority took over the costs of her maintenance care in September 1995. In October 1995 her father again went to court seeking for the ban on her identification to be lifted so that he could use publicity of the case to raise money for further treatment. Child B was revealed as Jaymee Bowen, and much publicity was forthcoming.

The media

Most people were aware of the Child B case only because it was reported by the media, and most of the information they gained about the case came from television, radio, or newspapers. The media ensured that the case was brought into a wider public arena and was something that people thought about. The ways journalists, editors, and producers chose to include or exclude, and place different emphases on, particular aspects of the case are likely to have contributed to people's attitudes about it.

The British media are not homogeneous. They have different target audiences and vary quite strikingly in their content and style. Although most national newspapers claim officially to be independent in terms of their political view, popular perception and academic analysis confirm that most national newspapers align themselves with a particular political party[1] and show explicit, but not necessarily total, support for that party's programmes and policies. Of the newspapers included in this study, the *Daily Mail* and *Daily Telegraph*, together with their Sunday equivalents, are most strongly aligned with the Conservative party. The *Daily Express* and the *Sun* also tend to support the Conservative party line but have been vocal in their dissent on particular issues and not reluctant to express opposing views. The *Guardian*, *Observer*, and *Daily Mirror* have more left wing ideological stances, which tends to mean support for Labour party policies, although this is not inevitable. It is interesting to note in the context of this study that the *Daily Mirror* has, in recent years, energetically reported incidents such as ward closures and patients being kept waiting, which can be seen as indicating deterioration within the NHS, presenting them as examples of the failings of the current Conservative government. The *Independent* has striven since its inception in 1986 to remain free of political allegiances.

Outline of study methods

In December 1995 we decided to identify important dates in the Child B case and to examine systematically the content of a broad range of media outlets on those dates. Our study was therefore retrospective, and our date sample was purposefully chosen. Our media sample comprised four tabloid (*Daily Express*, *Daily Mail*, *Daily Mirror*, and *Sun*) and four broadsheet (*Daily Telegraph*, *Guardian*, *Independent*, and *Times*) national newspapers, together with their Sunday equivalents; BBC and ITN news and current affairs programmes; 10 women's magazines; the *British Medical Journal*, *Health Service Journal*, and *Economist* (the *Economist*, however, did not cover the Child B case and is not discussed further here). For practical reasons the national newspapers were studied in more detail than the other media. Time and resources prevented us from formally including radio and satellite and cable television channels in our study, although we are aware that these represent important media sectors and that they did cover the Child B case. A preliminary investigation of BBC Radio 4 news and current affairs programmes showed that they were broadly similar in tone and in terms of people interviewed to BBC television programmes. Our pragmatic decision not to study these additional media outlets was guided by the suspicion that we were unlikely to cover different issues by studying them so the costs of including them were unlikely to be justified.

We identified key dates in the Child B case by considering press releases supplied by Cambridge and Huntingdon Health Commission, searching full text databases of the *Guardian*, *Independent*, and *Times* on CD ROM, and hand searching the *Daily Mail* and *Sun* newspapers from 10 March to 31 December 1995, inclusive. A summary of the key dates in the case is given in box 1.

Box 1 Key dates in the Child B case

9, 10 March	High Court hearing: Justice Laws ruled Cambridge Health Authority must reconsider whether to fund treatment
10 March	Court of Appeal hearing: High Court ruling overturned. Cambridge Health Authority said to have acted rationally and fairly. Ruled that courts should not decide such cases
11 March	Family accepted donation of £75 000 to fund treatment
13 March	Child B admitted to Portland Hospital
14 March	Child B commenced chemotherapy
2 April	Dr Gravett announced that tests to assess the effects of the chemotherapy and determine the course of future treatment would be carried out soon
4 April	Dr Gravett announced that the chemotherapy had not been successful enough to warrant a second bone marrow transplant. He would give Child B donor lymphocyte infusion treatment
29 April	Virginia Bottomley praised the health authority's handling of the case

continued

4 May	Dr Gravett announced Child B was in remission
5 August	Child B's birthday
21 August	Cambridge and Huntingdon Health Commission announced they were discussing future funding of Child B's care with her father
11 September	Cambridge and Huntingdon Health Commission took over responsibility for funding all Child B's maintenance care
25 October	High Court ruled Child B could be named so her father could use publicity to raise money. She is revealed as Jaymee Bowen
26 October	*Panorama* programme on Child B case transmitted in prime time, BBC1

One issue of each newspaper was searched on 10–15 March; 3–5 and 30 April; 3–5 May; 5 and 22–23 August; 11 September; and 25–27 and 29 October 1995. All issues of the specialist journals published between March and December 1995 were scanned, and the editors of 10 women's magazines were contacted and asked to supply details of any articles they had published about Child B. Print media articles were included in the study if they were primarily about the Child B case or if they were about a relevant issue or a related case and were printed as part of a spread of articles about Child B. An article was defined as a discrete portion of text with its own headline or appearing in a clearly identifiable box.

Television programmes were identified with the help of the information services of the relevant channels. If very similar news items had been broadcast on several different news programmes on the same channel, only one version (usually the longest one from the latest news programme of the day) was obtained and included in the study unless significant variations in subject matter could be identified from the information supplied. An item was defined as the portion of a programme about the Child B case. By definition, there could be only one item a programme, but this might include statements read by a presenter, interviews with various people, and film footage of different scenes.

We created a database of relevant print media articles and broadcast items. We examined the coverage of particular aspects of the case qualitatively by systematically going through each article or item and noting relevant quotations or points for consideration. All the quotations and points deemed relevant to each aspect of interest were then analysed, and care was taken to identify what was typical and what was exceptional. In presenting our findings we have tried to indicate whether quotations were selected to illustrate common features of reporting or a range of reporting types.

We present the results of the study of national newspapers first, providing an overview of coverage and consideration of: the editorial positions of the different newspapers; the different arguments which contributed or might have contributed to the decision about Child B's treatment; the roles of different players in making decisions about treatment; other cases reported in connection with the Child B case; and the "authorised knowers" quoted. Separate descriptions of the coverage of the case by television, women's magazines, and specialist journals then follow.

An overview of national newspaper coverage

National newspapers devoted a lot of prominent space to the Child B case, particularly in March 1995 around the time of the court hearings about whether the health authority was legally obliged to fund the treatments that her father wanted and the private donation that enabled her treatment to commence and then in late October 1995 when Child B's identity was revealed and a BBC television documentary on her case was transmitted.

The case made main front page news and was the subject of editorial comment in all the national newspapers studied in the period 10 to 15 March 1995. It also attracted "in depth" coverage, with most newspapers publishing spreads of articles reporting on various aspects of the case. These included Child B's medical and life history; her father's encounters with medical professionals and health service managers; the characters of the various players and their different perspectives on the case; leukaemia and its treatment; and how decisions about treatments and funding are, or should be, made. Stories about other people with leukaemia or other conditions for which new or expensive treatments represented a last resort were also reported in connection with the Child B case, and the *Daily Mirror* and *Sun* newspapers, which both "adopted" her cause, ran appeals to raise money for leukaemia research. For the six day period from 10 to 15 March 1995 inclusive, a total of 149 articles were identified in the eight national newspapers studied (including 21 in the Sunday newspapers of 12 March).

On 26 October 1995 Child B's story again made front page news on all the newspapers studied except the *Daily Express*, and over the next few days various aspects of the case were reported and commented on. Several articles at this time drew quite heavily on a BBC *Panorama* programme about Child B (revealed as Jaymee Bowen) which was transmitted in prime time on 26 October. The news that Child B's father was threatening to sue the health authority was reported in all the newspapers except the *Daily Express*, and some of the broadsheets considered the case in connection with a conference on health care rationing. Most of the newspapers at this time included some kind of reflection on the implications of Child B's survival to date.

Broadly speaking, in keeping with what is generally accepted about newspaper styles, the tabloids devoted more attention to the character and day to day life of Child B and her family (the human interest aspects of the story). Whereas the broadsheets were more inclined to consider the general issues that her case raised at greater length. The broadsheets by no means ignored human interest angles in their reporting, however, and the tabloids, particularly the *Daily Express* and *Daily Mail*, did discuss some of the issues raised by the case. Tables 5.1 and 5.2 show the number of articles of different types that appeared in daily national newspapers over the peak periods.

Table 5.1 Numbers of articles on news pages, leader articles, letters, features, and column pieces that met inclusion criteria between 10 and 15 March 1995 (excluding 12). The last two columns give total number of articles and total number of pages on which the case was mentioned during this period

	News	Leader articles	Letters	Column	Feature	Total articles	Total pages
Daily Express	10	1	0	0	0	11	6
Daily Mail	8	1	0	1	0	10	8
Daily Mirror	21	2	1	1	1	26	22
Daily Telegraph	18	1	2	0	1	22	10
Guardian	10	1	5	1	0	17	10
Independent	7	1	1	0	0	9	6
Sun	8	3	0*	1	0	12	7
Times	16	1	1	0	3†	21	12

* Fax messages of support from readers were printed alongside a news article on 13 March.

† Two law reports in the *Times* were recorded in the feature articles category.

Table 5.2 Numbers of articles on news pages, leader articles, letters, features, and column pieces that met inclusion criteria between 25 and 28 October 1995

	News	Leader articles	Letters	Column	Feature	Total articles	Total pages
Daily Express	2	0	0	0	0	2	1
Daily Mail	4	1	0	0	0	5	6
Daily Mirror	6	1	0	0	0	8	9
Daily Telegraph	5	0	0	1	0	6	5
Guardian	3	1	1	0	0	5	5
Independent	6	0	0	0	1	7	6
Sun	4	1	0	1	0	6	7
Times	5	0	0	0	1	6	6

Editorial stances in national newspapers, 10 to 15 March 1995

We focus first on editorial articles about Child B because they can be assumed to represent the dominant attitudes of newspapers towards the decisions made in the case and because they highlight the issues that newspaper editors thought warranted particular comment. The national newspapers adopted strikingly different editorial stances, varying particularly in the extent to which they focused on clinical or financial issues and in their judgments about the correctness of the health authority's decision not to fund further treatment. They also interpreted the significance of the case in a range of ways. For the most part, the basic positions adopted in editorial articles were reflected in the news reporting of each paper. Although opposing viewpoints were included in most newspapers, these tended to be marginalised, appearing on letters pages, in columns, or as other first person opinion pieces. Editorials in the *Daily Mirror* and *Sun* seemed to start from the position that Child B "needed" treatment and found it wholly unacceptable that she would not be given it by the NHS. They presented the health authority's decision not to fund the treatment as quite simply wrong and implied that it had been reached because financial considerations had been allowed to dominate. Box 2 gives a selection of quotations which illustrate their position.

The *Mail on Sunday* also talked about the "treatment she needs", although it acknowledged that "doctors counselled against it". Its

Box 2 The *Daily Mirror* and *Sun* condemned the decision

Headline: Condemned by bank balance. (*Sun*, 11 March)[2]

"What state is this country in when a girl's right to life hinges on the size of a hospital bank balance?" (*Sun*, 11 March)[2]

"The idea that the medical judgment of a health authority can be clouded by financial considerations is distasteful and obscene". (*Sun*, 11 March)[2]

Headline: A price too high to pay. (*Daily Mirror*, 11 March)[3]

"Money is everything in health care today. . . . A child's life now is worth only what a health authority's accountants are willing to pay for it". (*Daily Mirror*, 11 March)[3]

"Her father believes she was never treated as more than a name or number. No sick child should be seen as a mere statistic. If they are, health authorities will inevitably take decisions about them based purely on money". (*Daily Mirror*, 13 March)[4]

primary concern was "the scandal of waste and muddle headed priorities in the NHS".[5] The *Daily Mail* said that while everybody hoped Child B would get the treatment "she so desperately needs", which "might—just might" save her life, there was not enough money within the NHS for all treatments to be given.[6]

The broadsheet and *Daily Express* editorials were more inclined to acknowledge the complexity of the case and to start to debate some of the issues it raised regarding treatment and funding decisions. Relatively few editorial articles, however, explicitly considered the question of whether the treatment proposed for Child B was effective, appropriate, or in her best interests. Only five out of 16 editorial articles in the early period mentioned the possibility that the treatment might cause Child B more harm than good and/or acknowledged that the majority medical opinion had been that the proposed treatment was not the best course of action for her. Their main comments on this point are quoted in box 3. (The figure of five excludes the *Daily Telegraph*, which reported that "Doctors felt that the suffering she would undergo in the course of further treatment and the unlikelihood of her surviving it made the expenditure unwise"[7] but did not explicitly question whether the treatment would be in her best interests.)

Box 3 Questioning whether treatment was in Child B's best interests

"There seem to have been sound clinical reasons given for this refusal by the doctors responsible for her case. [They] were firmly opposed to the additional treatment, which they said would be experimental, not therapeutic and likely to cause great suffering. . . . While subjecting a dying child to needless futile suffering would strike most people as undesirable . . .". (*Times*)[8]

"The NHS doctors have decided enough is enough. Bone marrow transplants are debilitating operations. They concluded a second transplant had little chance of succeeding and opted instead for palliative care to allow the girl to enjoy a last few months of normal life". (*Guardian*)[9]

"Most of the consultants who have seen the child judge her chance of benefiting from further harrowing treatment to be slender. Others commenting on the case seem of the same opinion. But at least two are more optimistic about her chances of pulling through, or more inclined to feel treatment should be carried out however slight the chances of success. It is a difficult choice with no certain answers". (*Daily Express*)[10]

"Her plight highlights the fact that we now find it almost impossible to envisage that a child's life sometimes cannot be saved. . . . Sometimes parents and physicians fail to recognise when they should savour what is left of a child's life rather than trying to extend it further at a high cost to the child in terms of suffering". (*Independent*)[11]

"Before we are overwhelmed with indignation at the fate of Child B—'sentenced to death' according to one newspaper headline yesterday—we should recall the case of Laura Davies. . . . In all such cases, several questions are asked. Will treatment significantly improve the child's chances of survival? If the child does survive, will it enjoy an adequate quality of life? Can the suffering caused by the treatment itself be justified? And can the treatment be afforded?" (*Independent on Sunday*)[12]

The *Times* noted that the precise ground for the health authority's original decision not to fund further treatment for Child B was not clear, and commented that:

> "While subjecting a dying child to needless futile suffering would strike most people as undesirable, refusing treatment on the ground of cost is more difficult to accept."[8]

Other editorials seemed more certain that the issue of cost had played a part in the health authority's decision (the *News of the World* was the only one not to touch on costs). With the perhaps surprising exception of the *Daily Mirror*, they all discussed the Child B case at least once in the context of how money was spent within the NHS and/or how government funds were allocated to health care among other things.

The broadsheet editorials, with the exception of the *Daily Telegraph* and *Sunday Telegraph*, implicitly accepted that the concept of opportunity costs supported the argument for not treating Child B, assuming that the money could and would be spent on treatments which were more effective (or which would bring greater health gain and to more people) than the one proposed for her. The *Daily Express* explicitly stated:

> "Resources used on the little girl cannot be used on other cancer sufferers, including those whose chances of responding to treatment, and thus survival, are greater".[10]

The *Daily Telegraph* defended the health authority's decision as correct, but thought that:

> "Public understanding of this dilemma would have been better were the NHS not perceived as inefficient and bureaucratically arrogant. It is harder to defend the decision not to treat Child B when one hears of the spending spree on the administration of the NHS".[7]

In contrast, the other tabloids and the *Sunday Telegraph* editorials used the concept of opportunity cost in support of the argument that Child B should have been treated on the NHS. As box 4 illustrates, the treatment proposed for her was judged to represent a better use of money than other current expenditures in the NHS. There was a clear message in several editorial articles that the refusal to fund treatment for Child B would have been easier to accept if so much NHS money was not seen to be wasted or spent inappropriately on other things. For example:

"Why is it that there is never enough cash for what matters and always enough to spend on the fripperies?" (*Mail on Sunday*)[5]

Box 4 What editorial articles cited as examples of less worthy uses of NHS funds

- Administration and bureaucracy (*Mail on Sunday, Daily Telegraph, Sun*)
- Managers' cars (*Mail on Sunday, Sun*)
- Abortions (*Mail on Sunday, Sunday Telegraph*)
- Cosmetic surgery, especially breast implants (*Sun*)
- AIDS campaign (*Mail on Sunday*)
- Fraud by NHS staff (*Mail on Sunday*)

There were also a few suggestions that more money might be available for health care if it were not spent on other ("less appropriate") causes. The *Daily Mail* questioned the high priority given to the social security budget and welfare benefits,[6] while the *Independent* commented on expenditure on arms and unnecessary consumption.[11] The value judgments underlying comments about what was or was not worthy of funding were not explicitly acknowledged to be such in the editorial articles.

Several editorials noted the instinctive reaction of many people that Child B should be given treatment on the NHS. These findings were seen as reflecting widespread reluctance to accept that children sometimes die and a general sentiment that it is better to try something than do nothing. Box 5 illustrates some of these statements.

Box 5 Acknowledging people's immediate reactions

"Most people have no difficulty deciding whether B, the 10 year old Cambridgeshire girl dying from leukaemia, should be given the treatment that might just conceivably save her life. Of course she should. If there is even a remote chance of her beating the disease, so the argument goes, she should be provided with the necessary treatment . . .". (*Independent*)[11]

continued

"In a way that would have seemed incomprehensible to earlier generations, and would still seem so to the inhabitants of many Third World countries, we take a child's 'right' to life so much for granted that we regard an early death almost as a defiance of natural law. So when we are told that the National Health Service . . . has declined to spend £75 000 on an attempt to prolong a 10 year old's life, we are outraged. But . . .". (*Independent on Sunday*)[12]

"For any loving parent, the question raised in the Court of Appeal yesterday merits only one answer. Our children are beyond price. . . . Instinctively then, most of us know which side we're on in the dispute between Cambridge Health Authority and a father desperate to save his stricken 10 year old daughter. Though the little girl's chances of recovery are tragically slim, there is something profoundly shocking in the Authority's reluctance to spend £75 000 on a treatment which might—just might—save her life. Public dismay at last night's judgment is palpable". (*Daily Mail*)[6]

"There is not a parent in the land who does not feel for the father of the 10 year old girl dying of leukaemia. And no doubt the overwhelming majority would also, in their place, similarly fight to ensure every possible treatment is attempted. But neither the medical nor the moral issues involved are clear cut . . .". (*Daily Express*)[10]

The respective roles of medical skill and parents' wishes in decisions about whether or not to treat desperately ill children were briefly touched on by several editorials. The *Daily Mirror* and *Observer* both argued that parents should decide whether they wanted the child treated or not. The *Daily Mirror* noted that parents of children with life threatening illnesses "must listen to the advice of the doctors. They must weigh the chances of their child's survival. They must consider the effects of further painful treatment".[3] It then apparently forgot the fact that the advice of doctors in this case had been that further treatment was inappropriate because of its small chance of success and likely adverse effects and assumed that a necessary, beneficial treatment had been denied because of its cost.

The limitations of medical skill were touched on briefly by only two editorial articles. The *Daily Express* pointed out that there was not a complete consensus among medical professionals in Child B's case,[10] while the *News of the World* commented that doctors are not infallible.[13] Sympathy and admiration for the decision of Child

B's father to oppose the health authority (contesting the judgment of doctors who had been treating Child B) was expressed by several editorials. The question of how, to what extent, and in what circumstances people should listen to and accept doctors' advice was not explicitly critically considered.

The issue of who should be making decisions about health care rationing was raised in several broadsheet editorials. The *Daily Telegraph* insisted "It is right that doctors should determine who benefits because they have clinical expertise".[7] The *Guardian*, *Independent*, and *Observer*, on the other hand, advocated greater public involvement, as illustrated in box 6.

Box 6 Advocacy of public involvement in health care rationing decisions

"There are three key groups in the process: medics, managers and ministers. All have to play their part, even if ministers insist on calling it 'priority setting' rather than rationing. But the public too must be involved". (*Guardian*)[9]

"The only way forward is a more transparent and accountable NHS ... in which ordinary people play their part in setting priorities. This would mean that none of us could shirk responsibility for harsh choices". (*Independent*)[11]

"Health priorities deserve an open public debate". (*Independent on Sunday*)[12]

"The ministry must start laying down guidelines as to how these decisions are reached. It also has to promote the structures which both involve the public in the decision making and allow appeals for particular cases". (*Observer*)[14]

The *Guardian*, *Independent*, *Observer*, and *Times* all noted that rationing decisions had been made before this case but they had previously been made secretly by doctors. The move to greater openness about decisions on health care funding was explicitly welcomed by all except the *Observer*, which expressed some uncertainty about its benefits.

The political implications of the case were commented on by several editorials. The *Daily Mirror* and *Sun* saw it as an indicator of the current sorry state of the NHS and the government:

> "That is what the health service has been reduced to". (*Daily Mirror*)[3]

> "What state is this country in when a girl's right to life hinges on the size of a hospital bank balance? . . . If she dies because cash came first, there will be a national outcry that will rock this government and its health reforms to the foundations". (*Sun*)[2]

The *Observer* pointed out that the public expects the health minister to take responsibility or at least be answerable for incidents in which people's health suffers because of rationing decisions. The *Daily Telegraph*, which also referred to a report about NHS expenditure on bureaucracy, noted that:

> "Virginia Bottomley, the health secretary, . . . must take action to reassure the public that the NHS is being run for their benefit. If she does not, defensible clinical decisions will increasingly be portrayed as unjustifiable failures to set the right NHS priorities. Were that to happen, the danger to Mrs Bottomley would be beyond treatment". (*Daily Telegraph*)[7]

Box 7 summarises our understanding of the positions adopted in editorial articles about the health authority's decision not to fund further treatment for Child B. It is interesting to note that the *Daily Telegraph* thought ahead to the possibility that Child B might survive despite the poor prognosis she was given and commented that it would be inappropriate to alter judgments on the correctness of the health authority's decision in hindsight:

> "Now that a private benefactor has put up the money for her treatment, we sincerely hope that Child B's prognosis is proved wrong and that she recovers. But in the happy event of her doing so, that should not make the slightest difference to the soundness of the decision the health authority, acting on the best clinical advice, took in her case". (*Daily Telegraph*)[7]

Box 7 Position of newspaper editorials on health authority's decision not to fund treatment

Daily Express—Non-committal. There is a moral dilemma. There is no certain answer to the question of whether Child B would benefit from treatment. The issue of treatment cost cannot be ignored

Daily Mail—Non-committal. The decision was instinctively shocking, but sometimes decisions between patients will have to be made

continued

Mail on Sunday—Implied the decision was wrong. Money in the NHS is wasted on fripperies

Daily Mirror—The decision was wrong. It was based purely on money

Daily Telegraph—The decision was sound. . . . However, it would be better understood if the NHS did not waste so much money

Sunday Telegraph—Implied the decision was wrong. It caused understandable anguish. Less NHS money should be spent on abortions (death) and more on last chances of life

Guardian—Implied the decision was right. The case is emotional, but "a rational health service is as important as a national health service"

Independent, *Independent on Sunday*—The decision was difficult. Sometimes it will not be appropriate to give last chance treatments which cause suffering to children

Observer—Implied the decision was wrong. Parents' views should dominate. Although hard decisions must be made, people want them to be made with sympathy and understanding, not on the crude market principle. Most people would have said in this case let her have the treatment

Sun—The decision was wrong. It reflects an inappropriate emphasis on money in the NHS and inappropriate priorities in terms of NHS expenditure

News of the World—Ambiguous. Took the position that it was a good thing that Child B would get treatment, and argued that all parents would understand and admire B's father's actions. On the other hand, argued that life and death decisions should be made by doctors

Times—The grounds for the decision were unclear. If it was a decision not to subject a child to needless futile suffering, it was appropriate, but cost considerations have confused the issue

Editorial stances in national newspapers, 25–29 October 1995

Four newspapers (*Daily Mail*, *Daily Mirror*, *Guardian*, and *Sun*) discussed the Child B case in leader articles in the period immediately after the ban on her identification was lifted. All were broadly consistent with their earlier editorial stances. In particular, the *Daily Mirror* maintained its position that the health authority's decision had been purely financial and repeated its assertion that "money is all that matters in the health service".[15] The *Daily Mail* used the case to complain about wastage of public resources, and the *Guardian* stressed "We all have a vested interest in an efficient and fair health service".[16]

Three tabloid editorials praised Jaymee Bowen's character and determination to live and held her up as an exemplar, although to make different points, as shown in box 8.

Box 8 Tabloid editorials, 26 October 1995

"**What a girl!** . . . Whatever the rights and wrongs of whether the NHS should have paid for Jaymee's treatment, Jaymee's courage is an example to us all". (*Sun*)[17]

"**Jaymee's lesson to us all** . . . She has sophistication and insight well beyond her years. She has bravery which any adult would envy. But seeing and listening to her for the first time is not only revealing about her. It exposes even more the appalling decision by her local health authority to withhold the treatment which would save her life". (*Daily Mirror*)[15]

"**Public waste and a child's will to live** . . . At an age when, mercifully, most children have little sense of mortality, her words are unbearably moving: 'Never give up hope unless you are just on the last drop of life you have left'. This child's will to live rebukes the worries of the passing day and renders absurd the waste and extravagance of the state". (*Daily Mail*)[18]

The *Guardian* editorial commented on the Child B case in connection with a conference on rationing, which it had reported on its front page. It saw the case as "merely the most dramatic example of an issue which defines the problems of the health service", a graphical illustration that no matter what proportion of public expenditure is devoted to health care, rationing decisions will still have to be made.[16]

General newspaper reporting—the basic story

Between 10 and 15 March 1995 all the newspapers recounted the history of Child B's illness and treatment in one form or another, ranging from brief summaries provided as background to news reports to dedicated articles occupying half a tabloid page or more. There were some discrepancies among these accounts. For example, the terminology used to describe the different types of cancer Child B had had varied both between and within newspapers, as illustrated in box 9. Although these discrepancies would possibly not be noticed by most newspaper readers, they might have been confusing for readers interested in comparing Child B's illness and treatment with that of others with leukaemia known to them.

Box 9 What exactly was wrong with Child B?

"The girl, . . . who has acute myeloid leukaemia, had a transplant last year. . . . It was the second time she had been stricken by cancer in her short life. She had developed non-Hodgkin's lymphoma in September 1990". (*Daily Mail*)[19]

"[When she was 5, she developed] Hodgkin's lymphoma, a rare cancer which breaks down the body's immunity to infection". (*Daily Mail*)[20]

"The girl . . . was diagnosed as suffering from acute lymphoblastic leukaemia five years ago . . . in December 1993 [she] was found to have developed acute myeloid leukaemia, a form more difficult to treat". (*Guardian*)[21]

[Sept 90] Aged just five years old, the girl is diagnosed as having Hodgkin's disease, a cancer of the lymph glands . . . [Dec 93] she is now dealt another blow when acute myeloid leukaemia is diagnosed". (*Daily Mirror*)[22]

"She had been successfully treated for non-Hodgkin's lymphoma with common acute lymphoblastic leukaemia, diagnosed when she was aged five". [Article refers to a relapse, but gives no other diagnosis] (*Daily Telegraph*)[23]

The tale of events leading up to Child B's father taking legal action against the health authority was also reported in various forms. A basic outline, itself derived from the newspaper reports studied, is given in box 10.

Box 10 Summary of events leading up to the court case

- Child B relapsed: the acute myeloid leukaemia returned
- Consultants at Addenbrookes Hospital told her father that there was nothing more they could do and that they expected Child B to live no more than 6 to 8 weeks
- Child B's father sought a second opinion from the Royal Marsden Hospital, where consultants confirmed the prognosis given at Addenbrookes and again said there was no effective treatment
- Child B's father did not accept these opinions and contacted experts in America, who were more optimistic about the possibility of treatment
- Child B's father contacted Professor John Goldman at Hammersmith Hospital. News reports about his response are conflicting. They vary from he was willing to treat Child B but had no bed available to he didn't recommend treatment himself but suggested to her father that Dr Gravett might be willing to have a go
- Dr Gravett agrees to treat Child B privately, at an estimated cost of £75 000
- Cambridge Health Authority, after taking medical advice on the case, refused to make an extra contractual referral for Child B. They will not pay for her treatment
- Child B's father seeks legal advice and challenges the health authority's decision in court

As reporting of the case continued there was also some confusion about what treatment Child B was given by Dr Gravett. For example, an article in the *Guardian* of 23 August 1995 noted that Child B was "making a remarkable recovery after undergoing a controversial bone marrow transplant and chemotherapy",[24] although earlier articles in the same paper had pointed out that she would not be given a second bone marrow transplant.

There were some very different constructions of the story in the press. The *Daily Mirror* and the *Sun*, which "adopted" Child B as their own particular cause, became committed to the position that the treatment given by Dr Gravett was the necessary and best course of action. This left little room for entertaining the possibility that the NHS doctors and health authority were anything other than wrong. These two papers tended to construct a story in which

Child B's father and the benevolent hero, Dr Gravett, saved her life despite the determination of callous, financially minded "health chiefs" to deny her treatment.

The *Daily Mirror* fully supported Child B's father's actions. It tended to cast the health authority as the main villain of the piece, emphasising its role in the decision to refuse further treatment and playing down the fact that the doctors who had been caring for Child B explicitly advised against more chemotherapy and a second bone marrow transplant. Its first main news article on the case said that:

> "Cambridge Health Authority had refused to treat the girl, claiming her chances of survival were so slim that the £75 000 cost would be better spent on other patients. Experts also claimed that treating the girl would only prolong her suffering". (*Daily Mirror*)[25]

The paper's characterisation of the health authority and its managers as foolish and hard hearted was reinforced by comments about Cambridge and Huntingdon Health Commission being formed by a merger on April Fool's day[26] (1 April) and Stephen Thornton complaining about noise from pool parties held to raise money for a local special school.[27]

In its recounting of "the story of little B" the *Daily Mirror* pointed out only that "Doctors at Addenbrookes and the Royal Marsden told her distraught parents that nothing more can be done" and attributed the refusal to treat solely to Dr Ron Zimmern, director of public health and policy at the health authority.[22] The *Daily Mirror* gave a lot of space to the viewpoints of Child B's father and emphasised incidents which indicated that he had been badly treated. One article criticised the way he had been sent a "brutally casual" letter from a consultant at Addenbrookes in a long brown envelope posted second class.[28]

The *Guardian*, in contrast, placed more emphasis on the recommendation which was agreed on by doctors at two well respected hospitals that "any attempt to treat the leukaemia would be improper"[29] and "could not be justified because of the low chance of success and the pain it would cause".[30] It published criticisms of the health authority as made by Justice Laws but also aired the Appeal Court's view of the efforts of Child B's father as misguided.

Subsequent newspaper articles varied greatly in terms of the aspects of Child B's story that they emphasised and the way they presented her progress, signs of health, and chances of survival. The sheer amount of attention given to the case in all newspapers, however, was striking: events such as a shopping trip to Harrods, her return to school, and her birthday attracted national newspaper coverage comparable with the attention given to celebrities, even though she remained anonymous until late October 1995.

Newspaper coverage of the decision about treatment

The questions debated in early 1995 about whether Child B should be given further chemotherapy and possibly a second bone marrow transplant and, if so, whether the NHS should fund it were highly complex. They could be viewed from various different perspectives, and a wide range of considerations could be brought to bear. In this section, we describe how the newspapers reported various factors which were (or arguably should have been) considered in the decision about Child B's treatment. Although they are considered separately for ease of discussion, we recognise that they are not considered in isolation during decisions on treatment and funding. In general, newspaper reports gave only a partial picture of what had been argued by whom in the period leading up to and during the court hearings. Their selective presentations meant that the basis of the decision was often unclear and some conflicting impressions were given.

The chances of success

One of the arguments that the health authority used to support its position that further chemotherapy and a second bone marrow transplant were not appropriate for Child B (and/or were not a good use of limited NHS funds) was that they had only a very small chance of success. The counterargument put forward by her father was that any chance of survival, however small, was worth taking. Newspaper articles varied in the extent to which they were in sympathy with these arguments. Beyond reporting differences of opinion, however, the difficulties of determining at which probability of a favourable outcome treatments "should" be given were rarely explicitly considered.

Although death could be presumed to be the unfavourable outcome, it was not always possible to tell from newspaper reports precisely what was meant by "success"—for example, whether it meant achieving remission, disease free survival at 2 years, or long term survival. Information about the probability of success was also often vague, and reports of claims that the chances of treatment success were, for example, "too slim" were not always accompanied by any quantitive estimates of these chances. The quantitive estimates of success which were reported ranged from 2·25% or 2·5% (usually attributed to the health authority or the NHS doctors treating Child B) through 10% or 10–20% (usually attributed to Dr Gravett, to whom an estimate of 1% was also occasionally attributed) to 18% or 30–60% (attributed to American experts). Some of the distinctions that were made—for example, between the probability of chemotherapy achieving remission and the combined probability of chemotherapy achieving remission and a bone marrow transplant working—might not have been readily understandable to some lay readers.

The broadsheets generally paid more attention to quantitive estimates of chances of success than the tabloids, but even they rarely considered the validity and reliability of these estimates. Reports generally neglected questions about the sources of the estimates or how they were arrived at. One rare exception, a news article in the *Times*, briefly noted that:

> "American studies show that those who relapse within six months of their first transplant have less than a 10 per cent chance of benefiting from a second one, but those who relapse at more than 9 months have a 10–20 per cent chance". (*Times*)[31]

In the same article, Dr Gravett was reported as saying that it was difficult to say which side of the fence Child B fell on because she relapsed at exactly nine months.

A feature in the *Independent* was unusual in hinting at the unreliability of estimates used in arguments about the case. It noted that the 2·5% chance of survival suggested by Child B's doctor in January was much disputed and that the 20–30% survival figure currently quoted for her prospects by Dr Gravett was drawn from the small sample of 52 people who had received donor lymphocyte infusion since it was invented.[32]

The accuracy and precision of estimates were rarely considered. Some uncertainty about the estimates may have been communicated when a range of probabilities was given or when they were explicitly said to be estimates, beliefs, or opinions. A few articles indirectly indicated uncertainty by reporting different estimates within the same article or noting differences of opinion between experts. Box 11 illustrates something of the range of statements made over the course of four days in the *Guardian.*

Box 11 Some estimates of success as reported in the *Guardian*

"Mr Pitt claimed the chances of success, using statistics provided by Peter Gravett ... were in the region of 2·25 per cent. Other figures quoted by Mr McIntyre, suggested the chances were slightly higher".[21]

"B's father consulted experts in Los Angeles and Orange County, in the United States. They suggested treatment might have an 18 per cent chance of success".[29]

"Dr Gravett, a Harley Street consultant haematologist likely to be treating the girl, yesterday put the chances of success at 10–20 per cent".[33]

"The specialist in charge of her care admitted yesterday there was only a 1 per cent chance overall of a successful outcome. ... 'There is a 10 per cent chance of the initial remission, then a 10 per cent chance of the transplant working. There is only a 1 per cent chance of a successful outcome ...' Dr Gravett said".[30]

The difficulties of extrapolating from data about the average effects of treatment among a group of people to estimate an individual's chances of a favourable outcome were largely ignored in newspaper reports. Most implicitly assumed that the probabilities quoted were applicable to Child B. Her grandfather and Dr Gravett were both occasionally quoted as arguing that her chances were better than most (or better than other doctors were saying) because of her positive attitude and her strong character. Dr Thomas Stuttaford, writing in the *Times*[34] and Celia Hall in the *Independent*[35] noted that her chances were poorer than those of others with her condition because her current illness had probably been induced by previous therapy and because her first bone marrow transplant had failed.

The chances quoted were most often presented in terms of absolute percentages of people receiving treatment for whom there would be a successful outcome. They were almost always presented in a positive frame (that is, as chance of survival rather than chance of death). It is interesting to note that there is some evidence to suggest that people are more likely to opt for toxic treatments with side effects if outcome probabilities are presented in a positive frame.[36]

The possible side effects of treatment

During the court case, the health authority argued that further aggressive chemotherapy would be "distressing" and "unpleasant" for Child B and might do her more harm than good. The father's counsel argued that the "significant" chance of survival offered by treatment made it unreasonable to argue it was not in her interest to be given the treatment on the grounds that it may be unpleasant (that is, he argued that the possibility of adverse side effects was outweighed by the chance of survival). Again, newspaper articles varied in the extent to which they sympathised with, or reported other viewpoints sympathetic to, these positions. For example, the *Daily Mirror* quoted Dr Gravett as saying that high dose chemotherapy "would be no more unpleasant than having no treatment at all".[37]

Reporting of the health authority's arguments and the court hearings rarely included any specific details of what the side effects of treatment might entail. Several newspapers, however, covered these in background articles about leukaemia and its treatment. In some, medical experts external to the case supplied the information. For example, Dr Jillian Mann, a paediatric oncologist from Birmingham Children's Hospital, explained that:

> "Intensive chemotherapy would mean that children were prone to infection, could develop bleeding such as nose bleeds, might find it difficult to eat, could vomit and could lose their hair. . . . Treatment was often intensive for the first six months, with long spells in hospital". (*Independent*)[35]

More detail about possible side effects was given as Child B began to receive chemotherapy, and some newspapers gave fairly detailed descriptions of what she was likely to experience. For example, in the *Daily Telegraph*, Dr Gravett commented on the minor short term risks and the journalist on the more serious long term risks of treatment:

> "Potentially, she could feel very sick. It's possible she could have complications like a sore mouth and diarrhoea if she got an infection. But drugs are a lot better these days and probably she won't be very unwell."

"Last night she was due to have pre-hydration treatment, when fluids are fed into the body to minimise the risk of damage to her kidneys when chemotherapy drugs are administered". (*Daily Telegraph*)[38]

Very few articles mentioned the possible risks to the proposed bone marrow donor, Child B's sister. One exception appeared in the *Daily Telegraph*, where Dr Gravett explained that the decision whether or not to proceed with a bone marrow transplant would depend on how well the chemotherapy had worked.

"If there is a transplant her sister will be the ideal donor, but there must be absolutely clear justification for doing it. Her sister will have a general anaesthetic and operation, which will mean some discomfort. It is not fair to put her through that unless there is some kind of benefit".[39]

As treatment progressed, reports suggested that Child B wasn't unduly distressed by side effects and possibly suffered less than most. On 15 March 1995, the day after Child B started to receive chemotherapy, five national newspapers reported that she was in good spirits and enjoying her food. Their comments were fairly typical of the style in which Child B's progress was reported in the respective papers, and are included in box 12.

Box 12 Chemotherapy didn't seem to upset Child B

"Dr Peter Gravett . . . said she had spent the afternoon telephoning her friends, watching videotapes and eating lunch. 'It doesn't look as though we have even taken the edge off her appetite', he said. . . . The cocktail of drugs given in chemotherapy normally causes nausea, diarrhoea and mouth ulcers but other drugs are given to counter these effects. Dr Gravett said the absence of ill effects so far in the girl suggested the dosages were right". (*Times*)[40]

"The leukaemia girl refused NHS treatment last week started her therapy yesterday at the private London Clinic in good spirits and with no loss of appetite, according to Peter Gravett, the doctor treating her. She was spending the time watching videos". (*Guardian*)[40]

"Dr Peter Gravett . . . said 'I found her sitting up in bed on the telephone to one of her friends, while simultaneously watching a video and ordering her lunches and dinners from a stack of menus for the next four or five days'". (*Daily Telegraph*)[39]

continued

Headline: Teddy in one hand, tv zapper in the other, B declares: I feel fine.
"Yesterday . . . little B was taking chemotherapy in her stride. Sitting up in bed drinking tea and watching cartoons, the ten year old girl stricken with leukaemia shrugged her shoulders and said 'I feel fine'" (*Daily Mirror*)[42]

Headline: Plucky Miss B's full of beans!
"Brave cancer girl Miss B had her first chemotherapy session yesterday—then tucked into fish fingers, chips and beans. The ten year old showed a healthy appetite despite having three powerful drugs pumped into her body. She also chose her hospital food for the rest of the week. Consultant Dr Peter Gravett, 48, said: 'She is ordering everything. The nurses are amazed by her appetite and very pleased with it. It has lifted the whole atmosphere. She has made her choices with great delight. She seems partial to burgers, custard and sticky puddings'". (*Sun*)[43]

In the later period of coverage there was little return to the issue of trading off the possible benefits of treatment against possible side effects. The original position of the NHS doctors, that "there was no chance of a cure and the risk of embarking on more very intensive treatment was that the child would spend weeks or even months in hospital" which was reasserted by Professor Ross Pinkerton on the *Panorama* programme, was reported only by the *Daily Mail.* In contrast, Child B's comment to the *Panorama* programme that she would "rather have gone through more suffering to live than not to go through anything and die" was quite widely reported.

The palliative care option

The NHS consultants who had been treating Child B advised that, given the aggressive and distressing nature of possible further treatment and its low chance of success, her best interests would be served by providing palliative care only. The health authority's solicitor argued in court that:

> "The alternatives are a course of distressing treatments with heavy side effects which in all probability she would not survive, or a palliative therapy which would at least enable her to enjoy several weeks or months of normal life prior to regression". (*Daily Telegraph*)[44]

The newspapers varied in their propensity to accept this. Some reported other views. The *Daily Mirror*[37] and *Independent* were among those which reported Dr Gravett's counter:

> "The options are not for a child to have a few weeks of normal life or to come into hospital to have several months of intensive treatment. She actually has not got a normal life at the moment and what she has got can only deteriorate".[45]

Other than by Dr Gravett, the judgment of the NHS consultants was questioned in very few articles. One exception was an article in the *Times* by Dr Thomas Stuttaford:

> "There is no evidence that a death from untreated leukaemia is likely to be appreciably easier than one from the complications of treatment. The determining factor in the comfort of any dying patient lies in the skill of the doctors and nurses looking after them". (*Times*)[34]

In some tabloid articles, it was clear that Child B's father thought death without treatment would be far worse. The *Daily Mirror* quoted him as saying:

> "If she's left the way she is without treatment, she'll deteriorate in the way that will cause her so much agony she'll be on morphine. She won't even be able to walk upstairs. She'll have to take doses even serious drug addicts wouldn't want. Her blood will become purely cancerous cells and the pain will come from within her bones. It will be a pain you and I could never understand and which a 10 year old child shouldn't have to". (*Daily Mirror*)[28]

Many newspapers articles did not explicitly mention palliative care and implied that the alternative to chemotherapy and a second bone marrow transplant was no care at all. Some phrases, particularly those used in the later period of reporting, might seem to suggest that the NHS would have done nothing to care for Child B.

The status of the proposed treatment

The fact that further chemotherapy and a second bone marrow transplant had not been shown to be effective in cases like that of Child B was considered by the health authority in coming to its decision. In a press statement, they said the decision had been made "in the light of Department of Health policy to fund expensive new treatments only if they have been shown to be effective".

The term "experimental" was used in the press statement to mean unproved. The treatment was described as being "of an experimental rather than an established nature", and "experimental rather than of proven benefit". In the High Court the description of the treatment as experimental was contested by Child B's family solicitor, who argued that it was unjustified given the estimates of success and the opinion of the doctor prepared to undertake it. Although the High Court judge accepted this argument, Sir Thomas Bingham in the Appeal Court accepted the health authority's claim that the proposed treatment had to be regarded as experimental because it "did not have a tried record of success" and was "at the frontier of medical science".[46] Several news reports quoted this statement.

Several newspapers also noted that the NHS doctors treating Child B told the court that the proposed treatment would be "experimental rather than therapeutic". The term "experimental" in some contexts seemed to carry negative connotations, as illustrated by the following comment in an article which questioned whether treatments were always in the best interests of the children treated:

> "[Laura Davies] spent virtually all her five years in pain, undergoing treatment that many called pioneering but which might better be described as experimental". (*Observer*)[47]

Interestingly, the one use of the term experimental which did not clearly appear in the early newspaper coverage was with the meaning "being given in the context of an experiment or clinical trial". This is discussed further below.

The logical implication of several news reports was that Department of Health policy (or Cambridge Health Authority's policy, if widely applied) of not funding unevaluated treatments meant that no new treatments could ever be introduced. This was commented on in a few articles and the argument made that "if we don't try, we won't learn". The father of an unexpected survivor of leukaemia was quoted in the *Sunday Express*:

> "Referring to the health authorities' argument that the treatment was experimental, he added: 'in 1975 they were all guinea pigs, but we have made tremendous progress in treating leukaemia' ". (*Sunday Express*)[48]

The possibility of contributing to research

Very few newspaper articles mentioned the argument that the treatment proposed for Child B might be justified if it was conducted as part of a research programme to evaluate its effectiveness and could therefore contribute to knowledge of how best to treat people with her condition. The *Guardian* was alone in reporting the health authority's solicitor as arguing that the only basis on which the treatment could be justified was for experimental or research reasons.[21] This argument did not appear in the law reports published in the *Times*.

Recent progress in rates of success of treatment for leukaemia was briefly referred to by several articles in the early period of coverage, but only the *Daily Mirror* devoted an article to leukaemia research (this included the logo of the "Daily Mirror B appeal" alongside its headline). The article attributed current cure rates in leukaemia to "brilliant research" and argued that it was only through further research that better combinations of drugs and ways to reduce their side effects would be found. It described how "the 20 major centres treating childhood cancer throughout Britain work together in the UK Children's Cancer Study Group" and argued that "co-ordinated research is essential" but made no mention of the facts, reported in a few other papers, that the group had advised against treating Child B and that she was being treated outside it.[49] The appeals organised by the *Daily Mirror* and *Sun* newspapers both at some point said that donations would be used for leukaemia research, but neither newspaper suggested that Child B could or should participate in such research.

The notion that the treatment of one person with a new technique could contribute to knowledge and improve the treatment of future patients was alluded to in a letter to the *Times* from the mother of a boy who had, despite some contrary medical advice, been given extremely expensive "state of the art" treatment for acute myeloid leukaemia and, against the odds, had survived. The letter concluded:

> "His treatment pushed back the frontiers of knowledge about this awful disease and furthered research which has helped other young patients". (*Times*)[50]

Few newspaper articles did anything to convey the limitations of knowledge gained by observing single patients or the importance of well designed clinical trials to evaluate effectiveness of treatment. An article by Polly Toynbee in the *Independent* provided the fullest consideration of the tension between the need for coordinated research and the desire to give last hope treatments to individuals.

She quoted Professor Clifford Bailey of the UK Children's Cancer Study Group as saying:

> "If we followed up every suggestion of a breakthrough without a proper trial, we would waste our energies on too many false starts". (*Independent*)[32]

This is a dying child! The imperative to do something

Child B's father believed that any small chance of survival should be taken. His view was endorsed by Justice Laws in the High Court, and it was widely acknowledged in the newspapers that there was general sympathy for the desire to try anything possible rather than to let a child die. The life or death nature of the case and the fact that it involved a child were played up, particularly in the tabloid reporting. Child B's age was mentioned in nearly all reports, and the *Sun* referred to her as "Little B" or "Little Miss B".

Some more considered pieces, particularly but not exclusively in the broadsheets, acknowledged the emotional pressures generated towards trying whatever possible treatment was available. Several articles argued that when all the risks, benefits, and uncertainties of the treatment were considered, the decision might need to be taken not to treat and to let a child die. They acknowledged, however, that this could be hard to accept. One journalist commented:

> "When a child falls ill with a potentially fatal illness, parents naturally wish to do everything possible and fear they will feel guilty later if they do not. There can be no hard rules about whether to intervene or let nature take its course. Each case must be judged on its own merits, but doctors have a moral responsibility to advise against treatment if it will only prolong suffering".[51]

However,

> "There is no chance that a second bone marrow transplant with further chemotherapy can cure relapsed myeloid leukaemia. If the treatment itself is not lethal, the few months it might bring will be complicated by grievous side effects. The question of funding for this treatment is irrelevant".[51]

The tendency to attach more sympathy to and be more inclined to treat a dying child was only rarely analysed in the newspaper coverage of the case. A couple of feature articles commented on discrimination against older people in terms of access to health care.

Health service resources are limited and treatments carry opportunity costs

That resources for health care are finite and health authority budgets limited was stated quite often in media coverage of the case. There were also some suggestions that more money should be devoted to health care, whether this be derived from general taxation, reductions in the salaries of health service managers, or diversion from other areas of public spending. In the early period of reporting, as mentioned above, the concept that money spent on one thing in the health service could not be spent on something else was widely used in newspaper articles but in two different ways. Some argued that the £75 000 which proposed treatment for Child B would cost could be better spent on more effective treatments for other patients, while others argued that money currently spent on other things in the NHS could be better spent on the proposed treatment of Child B. The irony of the costs of the court hearings being enough to pay for the contested treatment was not lost on some papers, several of which included small boxed articles itemising the legal bills incurred by the health authority.

Several articles adopted a moral high ground when discussing opportunity costs, viewing it as shameful that money could be spent on cosmetic surgery (implied to be unnecessary), treatment of people with AIDS (the amounts being deemed to be excessive and the beneficiaries undeserving), and administrative procedures (termed bureaucracy, with the attendant connotation that they were unnecessary) while an innocent child who was dying (seen as one of the most deserving of causes) was denied treatment. The *Sunday Express* devoted a whole article to this line of thought just one day after its daily counterpart had stressed in an editorial how the money requested for Child B's treatment could more effectively be used to help other cancer patients.[52]

The Child B case and health care rationing

Although there were serious doubts about the clinical appropriateness of the treatment that Child B's father fought for, her case was presented in the newspapers primarily as an example of health care rationing, and it triggered some discussion of the general issue of health care funding, particularly in the broadsheet newspapers. Most newspapers seemed to accept that rationing was inevitable, and several were keen to point out that rationing decisions were not a new phenomenon but that the public had simply not been aware of them until recently. Thus, for example, an anonymous former consultant haematologist was reported in the *Daily Telegraph* as saying that in the second world war a decision was made to use the limited available supplies of penicillin to treat syphilis rather than gangrenous wounds because more soldiers would be saved that way. He expected that "that would have caused a row if it was well known".[53]

One novel argument which assigned a positive value to health care rationing was introduced by Dr John Collee, the *Observer*'s regular medical columnist:

> "The point is that at some level we actually need the excuse of limited resources to protect us from the extremes of technological medicine". (*Observer*)[54]

Most other articles focused on the difficulties of rationing decisions and raised the questions of who should make them and how. Several newspapers cited people such as Philip Hunt, director of the National Association of Health Authorities and Trusts, who emphasised the need for clearer guidance at a national level about the processes and criteria used to decide which treatments should be funded for which people.

In the later period of coverage the *Guardian* and *Independent* explicitly linked the Child B case with a conference on health care rationing. The consensus of that conference had been that rationing would be inevitable, and very few newspaper articles considered the possibility that it was not. For the *Guardian*, the questions were not about whether rationing exists but about "what size of health service we can afford . . . and how transparent and democratic the decisions to ration should be".[16] In keeping with their editorial comments in the early period these newspapers claimed to be keen to see greater public involvement in difficult decisions about health care rationing.

The roles of doctors, parents, and children in treatment decisions

The Child B case did lead to some consideration in newspaper articles of the question of who should make decisions about the treatment of seriously ill children. The importance of both medical skill and the views of the family were stressed, and in many articles some form of shared decision making was implicitly advocated, although there was little practical advice as to what should be done when doctors and parents disagree, as happened in this case. Newspaper coverage of the Child B case very rarely mentioned that it is now NHS policy to promote patient choice in health care.

One of the apparently unusual features of the Child B case was that her father disagreed with the doctors who had been treating her, even after he had obtained a consistent second opinion. The rarity of the kind of explicit challenge to medical expertise which his actions represented, however, were scarcely commented on. The question of the extent to which such challenges are necessary or desirable is highlighted in the second part of this chapter. We note here that even in the early period of reporting there were signs that media coverage of the case could have the effect of reducing the trust that people put in doctors.

An article in the *News of the World* on 12 March 1995 featured the parents of a girl who had died of leukaemia after being treated at Addenbrooke's Hospital. They were said to be "tortured with guilt" after hearing of Child B's father's fight for further treatment for his daughter, and the father was quoted as saying:

> "I keep asking myself if they let Sharon die because of money as well. B's father had the guts to find out why they were stopping her treatment. I didn't. I never questioned it. I accepted it. But it makes me feel now that if I'd done what he's done would I have got the same answer, 'We can't afford it'? It's really bugging me. Did I let my daughter die without at least finding out what chance she had and what I could do about it . . . You accept what the doctors tell you because they are the experts and you trust them. Now I can't help asking if I did the right thing".[55]

Such comments also raise questions about the possible impact of the Child B case on the placebo effect associated with trust in health professionals. Possibly, if people have less confidence in the advice and treatment their doctors give they may be less likely to experience benefit from it. This was not covered in newspaper reports.

In general terms, the important role of medical advice was emphasised even by the *Daily Mirror*, the newspaper that most vehemently opposed the decision not to treat Child B. Although many reports of the case made it clear that doctors could have different opinions about things, there was little explicit consideration of how people might judge which doctors are right. Child B's father effectively didn't like what specialists at Addenbrookes told him nor what those at the Royal Marsden told him when he sought a second opinion. He kept asking until he found a doctor who would say that treatment was worth trying and was willing to carry it out. Whether this kind of search was admirable or misguided was not always clearly considered, although a few articles quite strongly took one stance or the other. The fact that people will probably always be able to find a doctor willing to provide the treatment they want as long as they have the money to pay to be treated privately was also occasionally referred to, but neither the possible harms nor the inequity of this attracted much comment.

The importance of children's views about their own treatment received a little attention from the newspapers. Justice Laws had said in the High Court that a 10 year old child could not make an informed decision as to whether it was in her best interests to undergo treatment or decline it so her parents had to take that decision for her.[56] In contrast, several people were reported in newspaper articles as arguing that Child B's wishes *should* be elicited and taken into account during the decision. They implicitly questioned whether Child B's father was necessarily acting in her best interests and argued that a child of 10 who had already received treatment for leukaemia probably would have her own opinions about further treatment. The general issue of the competence of children of various ages, particularly those who have experienced illness and treatment, to participate in treatment decisions and provide informed consent was not explored in the newspapers in connection with the Child B case.

It was argued at the time of the court hearings that since Child B apparently didn't know how seriously ill she was she couldn't be asked for her opinion. There were, none the less, some indications in early newspaper reports that Child B would have wanted the proposed treatment and the chance of life it was purported to offer. The *Daily Mirror* claimed an exclusive on 13 March 1995 for its front page story that Child B had heard about her own case on the radio, not knowing it was about her, and told her father that if she had been the girl she would have wanted treatment.[57] Several newspapers also reported that Dr Gravett had insisted that Child B be told how ill she was and (although this was less often reported) agree to further chemotherapy before he would treat her. The "news" that she was eager for treatment to start once she did know was widely reported and even made the front page of the *Times*.[58] Later newspaper coverage also picked up on the assertion Jaymee Bowen made on the BBC *Panorama* programme that if she had been asked at the time she would have said that she wanted treatment.

Newspaper portrayals of the NHS consultants and Dr Gravett

The newspapers varied in their characterisations of the NHS consultants who advised against further treatment for Child B and Dr Gravett who agreed to give it in the private sector. As noted above, there were some key differences in the way the story of Child B was constructed. The extremes of the roles into which Dr Gravett was placed by these constructions were the benevolent hero who stepped in to help a dying girl whom all others had abandoned (this was most obvious in the *Daily Mirror* and the *Sun*) and the unorthodox outsider, working in the private sector, who was more cavalier and less obviously respectable and well intended than most consultants (the clearest examples of this appeared in the *Independent*).

Box 13 Broadsheet descriptions of Peter Gravett

"Dr Gravett, 48, set up the bone marrow transplant unit at the London Clinic in 1985 after retiring from the Royal Army Medical Corps, in which he was a lieutenant colonel. He says he has performed 150 bone marrow transplants in the past ten years. He works only in private practice and is a consultant haematologist at the clinic". (*Times*)[31]

"Dr Peter Gravett, the private consultant who is expected to supervise the chemotherapy". (*Sunday Times*)[59]

"Dr Peter Gravett, the Harley Street consultant haematologist likely to carry out the treatment . . .". (*Times*)[60]

"Dr Peter Gravett, the private consultant whom patient B's parents want to carry out the treatment, said yesterday he disagreed with National Health Service doctors who said it was not worth the cost". (*Independent*)[45]

continued

"Dr Peter Gravett, a Harley Street consultant haematologist widely reported as likely to carry out the treatment...". (*Independent*)[61]

"Dr Gravett joined the army after qualifying in London. He rose to become a lieutenant colonel in the Royal Army Medical Corps and consultant haematologist at the Queen Elizabeth military hospital in London. He was honorary consultant at the now-closed Westminster Hospital before going into private practice, where he is well known for his work on bone marrow transplants. Dr Christine Costello, head of haematology at the Chelsea and Westminster Hospital, said Mr Gravett was 'very good'. She added: 'He is a good man for the job in hand'." (*Daily Telegraph*)[53]

In terms of direct descriptions of Dr Gravett the broadsheets were quite measured and tended to avoid explicit value judgments. They all provided similar information about his career history, as illustrated in box 13. The *Daily Telegraph* was the most positive and was the only paper to report a third party opinion on Dr Gravett's credentials. Among the tabloids, the *Daily Mirror* and *Sun*, in keeping with the role in which their story constructions placed him, described Dr Gravett in more obviously positive terms, as the quotations in box 14 show.

Box 14 Portrayals of Dr Gravett: *Daily Mirror* and *Sun*

"**This bed is ready NOW . . . just give me the chance to save her.** A Harley Street doctor said last night he was ready to start immediate treatment on the 10 year old leukaemia girl condemned to die in days. Pleading to be given the chance to help the stricken youngster, consultant Dr Peter Gravett said he disagreed with experts who said she was beyond help and would suffer if treated . . . Dr Gravett, 49, of the London Clinic, was contacted by the girl's desperate father after doctors at both Addenbrookes and the Royal Marsden told him nothing more could be done". (*Daily Mirror*)[37]

"Dr Gravett is the London based consultant sought out by the father of the girl". (*Sunday Mirror*)[62]

"She was given a general anaesthetic by a team headed by the top consultant Dr Peter Gravett". (*Daily Mirror*)[63]

continued

"Top doc gives cancer girl new hope as millions of *Sun* readers pray for a miracle: I'll start treatment to save little B's life today. . . . Harley Street specialist Peter Gravett said last night: 'We want to get on with it as soon as possible' . . . Dr Gravett, 49—who has a son aged 18—hopes to treat B at the London Clinic . . . Dr Gravett said 'We have performed four second bone marrow transplants at the London Clinic. We are very well equipped'." (*Sun*)[64]

Picture captions

"LIFE-SAVER: This is Dr Gravett and the £25,000 Cobe Spectra machine . . .". (*Daily Mirror*, 11 March)

TREATMENT: Dr Gravett. . . . REFUSAL: Dr Zimmern". (*Daily Mirror*, 11 March)

"MESSAGE OF HOPE: Dr Peter Gravett believes the delay has caused no harm to little B". (*Daily Mirror*, 14 March)

"Final hope . . . but consultant Peter Gravett is determined to give Miss B the best chance of survival". (*Sun*, 13 March)

The NHS consultants at Addenbrookes and the Royal Marsden who had treated Child B received less explicit newspaper attention. Their high calibre and standing was emphasised in some news reports, and the health authority's representatives (and others who agreed with their decision) cited the experience and good reputation of those who advised against further treatment. In contrast, those articles which emphasised the positive nature of Dr Gravett's role and which later on saw Child B's remission as vindicating the judgments of her father and Dr Gravett, inevitably implied shortcomings on the part of the NHS consultants.

In the early period of reporting none of the NHS consultants were directly quoted. The only NHS consultant who was identified was Dr Valerie Broadbent, who was criticised in an article in the *Daily Mirror* for the manner in which she informed Child B's father that her platelets were low.[28] Dr Broadbent was also praised in a *Sunday Mirror* article written by the father of another of her patients. In this she was described as "a totally dedicated doctor and ranked among the best in the country".[65] The author of this article emphasised that he could not believe that "if cost were the only consideration, Dr Broadbent would let any accountant or bureaucrat dictate treatment for 'her' cancer kids". He essentially argued that she would have acted as an advocate for treatment for Child B if she had thought that treatment was in her best interests.

Newspaper coverage of the decision to give donor lymphocyte infusion

In early April 1995 Dr Gravett announced that he would not be giving Child B her second bone marrow transplant but would treat her with donor lymphocyte infusion. He was widely quoted regarding the chances of success and possible side effects of this treatment, and most newspapers printed his justification for going ahead with what he admitted was "experimental" treatment. Given the publicly aired opposition from medical professionals within the NHS to the second bone marrow transplant which he had considered previously, his careful explanations of the rationale underlying his decision to offer donor lymphocyte infusion could have been intended to anticipate or counter criticism of his handling of the case. From the way quotations were reported it seems that on at least some occasions Dr Gravett's statements were made in response to journalists asking challenging questions:

> "The term 'guinea pig' could be applied to B, he conceded. But he went on: 'This is not desperation. If she were going to spend the next three months in hospital being really sick, I would agree it was something we should not continue with. But that is not the case' ". (*Daily Mail*)[66]
>
> "Dr Gravett accepted that Child B was, in effect a guinea pig for donor lymphocyte infusion . . . 'It is possible to justify that description, but unless we are prepared to use promising technology on patients who have no other option, we would never be able to develop new treatments', he said". (*Times*)[67]

In the event, although there was some scepticism about the likely effectiveness of donor lymphocyte infusion, no explicit criticism that it was being tried on Child B was reported in the newspapers studied during the April–May period.

Several newspapers reported the likely success rates of donor lymphocyte infusion, with the tabloids tending to present the more confident picture. Box 14 shows how its chances of success were reported in news articles. The unproved status of donor lymphocyte infusion received relatively more attention than the second bone marrow transplant had received around the time of the court hearings. Reports which described donor lymphocyte infusion as the experimental treatment being given to Child B *instead of* a second bone marrow transplant may have implied that second bone marrow transplants were quite orthodox. The term experimental continued to be used in connection with donor lymphocyte infusion to mean "of unproved benefit" and continued in some newspapers to carry negative connotations. The term "pioneering" was used in more enthusiastic reports.

Box 15 What chances did donor lymphocyte infusion offer?

"Dr Gravett admitted he did not have full figures about the success rate of the experimental treatment he is proposing, but said two of the seven patients he had heard of receiving the treatment had gone into remission. A spokeswoman for the Imperial Cancer Research Fund said the idea of using donor defence cells to attack leukaemia was highly experimental and the success rates were not known". (*Guardian*)[68]

"Dr Gravett said he was aware of seven cases in Europe in which the transfusion treatment had been used. Two had gone into complete remission, two had partial remission, and in the others there had been no response. Professor John Goldman of the Hammersmith Hospital in west London, who pioneered the donor injection treatment three years ago, said that once the therapy started, there was a 30 to 50 per cent chance of the girl recovering". (*Times*)[67]

"Dr Gravett admitted that B could be seen as a 'guinea pig', but said results with the new treatment were encouraging". (*Daily Mirror*)[69]

"Success rates have been high on both sides of the Atlantic. Twenty patients recently treated in a New York clinic all went into complete remission. Among seven patients treated in Europe, two went into complete remission, two went partially into remission, and three had no response. Professor John Goldman, who began using DLI at Hammersmith Hospital three years ago, said '. . . The chances of remission in patients with a similar rare form of cancer to Child B are 30 to 50 per cent, and up to 80 per cent in others' ". (*Daily Express*)[70]

"The technique . . . is still very much at the experimental stage. But of 20 chronic myeloid sufferers receiving the treatment in New York, all had gone into remission, Dr Gravett said". (*Daily Mail*)[66]

The identification of Child B as Jaymee Bowen

In the early stages of the case, when he was challenging the health authority's refusal to fund further treatment for Child B in court, her father applied for a court order to prevent her from being publicly identified to protect her from the knowledge of how ill she was. He later sought to have that court order lifted so that he could attract more publicity for her case to raise money for any future treatment she might need. The ban was lifted on 25 October 1995, and Child B was revealed as Jaymee Bowen.

The reluctance of the Appeal Court judge who heard the case to lift the ban on identifying Child B was reported in several newspapers:

> "I greatly regret the necessity to exploit the medical problems of this child for financial gain. . . . But I don't think the maintenance of reporting restrictions can be justified if the consequence were the denial of treatment which might be therapeutic and life saving". (*Independent*)[71]

The *Guardian* commented on the embarrassment which this decision (particularly, one presumes, the rationale said to underly it) caused for the health authority. Child B's survival to date was inevitably seen in some newspaper articles as not only a vindication of her father's determination to secure treatment but also as confirmation that the doctors who gave a gloomy prognosis and said nothing further could be done were wrong and that the health authority acted inappropriately when it refused to fund her treatment. Reflection on the complex implications of her case was largely limited to the broadsheet newspapers.

Meanwhile, the lifting of the identification ban marked a new stage in the entry of Jaymee Bowen into the world of major media celebrities. With the exception of the *Daily Express* she featured on the front page of every national newspaper studied on 26 October 1995. All seven articles drew heavily on a BBC *Panorama* programme about Child B which was transmitted that evening. The newspapers focused on the human interest side of the story, including Jaymee Bowen's character and her current state of health and activity. The quotations from Jaymee which attracted the most newspaper attention were those emphasising that if she had been asked at the time she would have said would want the treatment which offered her a chance of life, even if it involved suffering; that she was determined not to give up; and that if she met the chief executive of the Cambridge Health Authority she would go over and "whack him one".

Other cases reported in connection with the Child B case

The stories of quite a range of other patients were reported in both broadsheet and tabloid newspapers in connection with the Child B case. They fell into four broad categories: people who had survived leukaemia and other conditions after being given a fatal prognosis; people who had decided against further treatment for themselves or a seriously ill child; children who had been treated ouside the NHS after NHS doctors advised that no further treatment was possible; and children who had been denied NHS funding for a particular treatment.

The mother of a boy who had defied his prognosis and survived after they had searched for a consultant willing to treat him actively wrote a letter to the *Times* to tell his success story and ended up appearing on the front page under the headline, "Hope for Girl B after survival of boy 'not worth treating'".[72] Among other unexpected survivors of childhood leukaemia whose stories were published was Neil Collier, who, contrary to doctors' predictions of 20 years ago, was not only alive but the father of a family. He argued in the *Sunday Express* that "any patient facing death would tell doctors 'Give me all the treatment you've got and I don't care how much it hurts'".[48]

That some people disagree and prefer not to undergo all possible treatment was exemplified in the *Daily Telegraph* by Gunilla Easton, whom the case of Child B "prompted to present the other side of the debate".[73] When told that several operations had not been successful in removing all of her brain tumour, she and her husband decided not to spoil the last few months they had together by being tied to hospital chemotherapy schedules. The *Daily Telegraph* also explained in another article how Chris Irwin had decided that death was a more humane option than a third liver transplant for her 5 year old daughter. The article noted that Mrs Irwin had never regretted her decision but pointed out that in her case no one suggested the operation could not be afforded.[74]

The *Sunday Mirror* published an article by the father of an 8 year old boy with non-Hodgkin's lymphoma who was being treated by the same consultant at Addenbrooke's Hospital as Child B. It was headlined “My son is ill—but I disagree with B’s dad” and described some of the difficulties he has faced as a result of his son’s illness. The article praised the consultant concerned, emphasising that the author believed the decision not to treat Child B further was made by doctors “dedicated to beating cancer in children” on the grounds of the unlikely success and severe side effects of further treatment and said he didn’t believe Child B’s father was right to fight the decision.[65]

Several cases were presented of children who had been treated outside the NHS (often in America) after British doctors had advised nothing further could be done. Some of these stories, particularly on the tabloid pages, might have had the effect of bolstering the argument that there was hope that Child B could survive and therefore should be treated. They might also have given the impression that British doctors do not know as much as American doctors, that they do not try as hard as they might, or that the NHS is “failing” sick children.

The case of Laura Davies was used in several different ways in connection with the Child B case. Laura had various major disorders of the digestive system, and when it got to the stage that her only chance of survival was a multiorgan transplant, British doctors advised that nothing more could or should be done. Her parents raised funds for surgery in America, however, and Laura lived through several major operations before dying in November 1993. The *Daily Mirror* had a photograph of Laura under the headline “Message of hope” and printed a message from Laura’s family to Child B’s parents urging them not to give up. Laura’s grandmother was quoted as saying the government were denying treatment to Child B which could be offered in this country, from which it could be inferred that she thought Child B should be given the treatment.[75]

Several broadsheet papers also referred to Laura’s case but used it to suggest that further treatment for Child B might be inappropriate. They emphasised the surgical ordeals Laura had been put through and raised questions about how the best interests of a child in such situations could be determined. The *Independent of Sunday* suggested that in Laura’s last months even her parents had second thoughts about their decision to go ahead with the treatment.[12] The *Guardian* reported that, “It was argued then that her best interests had not been considered, and that there were grounds for setting up multi-disciplinary teams, with someone other than the parents acting as advocate of the child".[76] Dr John Collee, writing in the *Observer*, recalled a number of cases of children "whose treatment has been expedited by public appeal" and expressed concern about the extremes of technological medicine. He argued:

> "When a nurse or a doctor tells you that an operation is not worth it, they are generally not talking about the expense. They mean it's not worth the suffering . . . The media appeal can be a dangerously powerful instrument. It's being used more and more as a way of taking medical decisions out of doctors' hands and putting them into the public domain. Unfortunately certain important details of the case tend to be lost in the translation".[54]

One case that was widely reported in national newspapers in connection with the Child B case involved a health authority resisting an NHS doctor's request for funding for an expensive treatment for a child in his care. Gavin Gerrard's doctor thought it was worth trying a drug called DNase to see if it would improve his condition (he had cystic fibrosis). Northumberland Health Authority, however, was refusing to pay for it, saying it was not known to be effective, so his parents were preparing for legal action.

Authorised knowers

A fairly wide range of people and organisations were used as "authorised knowers" by the newspapers to comment on various aspects of Child B's story. Her family (with the exception of her mother, who had apparently left the family when Child B was a toddler) and school teachers were called on to describe her character and day to day life. The then health secretary, Virginia Bottomley, was extensively quoted early on in the case reaffirming how important it was that clinical decisions were made by doctors, supporting the health authority's decision, and expressing sympathy for Child B's family. Other politicians were also occasionally quoted, particularly those who asked questions about the case in the House of Commons.

The opinions of medical and health service management organisations such as the BMA and NAHAT were widely reported, and a range of professors of paediatric oncology and haematology supplied background information or commented on issues raised by the case. GPs and public health practitioners, on the other hand, were not quoted in connection with the case. People with experience of having to make decisions about the treatment of their seriously ill children or themselves were also recognised as having viewpoints which warranted attention, as mentioned above. One group which was noticeably not given a voice was that of religious and spiritual leaders or representatives.

What the newspapers saw the Child B case as highlighting

The newspapers varied in the way they reported the Child B case and also in what they saw it as illustrating or signifying. Explicit comments about the importance of the case were more common in the broadsheet press than the tabloids. Box 16 illustrates the types of comments made in the period immediately after the lifting of the ban on identifying Child B, at a time when she was out of hospital and in remission. The focus was very much on the rationing of health care and the remarkable personality of Jaymee Bowen. The uncertainties of medicine and the difficulties of decisions about how to treat seriously ill children, particularly when the only possible treatments have not been evaluated, were not emphasised by the newspapers at this time.

Box 16 What the Child B case highlights

"From now on, she will be a cause celebre, the famous embodiment of the nation's obsession with where to set the limits of public health care; and while she will be hailed as the epitome of courage, a battler who is seemingly overcoming the pessimism of the NHS authorities, the reality is that her life has become public property". (*Daily Telegraph*)[77]

"Cases like that of Child B have exposed the lack of clear guidelines for authorities when many experts are warning that demand for health care, and its rising costs, are outstripping available resources". (*Guardian*)[78]

"The controversy this week over [Child B] is merely the most dramatic example of an issue which defines the problems of the health services. The real argument is not whether rationing exists.

continued

It is what size of health service we can afford, within which rationing operates, and how transparent and democratic the decisions to ration should be". (*Guardian*)[16]

"However long she lives, the image of Jaymee Bowen will linger in the nation's psyche. Her loving and determined father has made sure of that by thrusting her so skilfully into the spotlight . . . the 11-year-old who was named last week as Jaymee Bowen has touched millions of hearts. . . . For most of us, however, Jaymee's story is an entirely emotional one". (*Observer*)[47]

"The Child B story has already generated a lively debate on the rationing of health care, the split between purchaser and provider in the NHS, and the future of experimental treatment". (*Times*)[79]

Television

The Child B case was given prominent coverage on national terrestrial television news and current affairs programmes, particularly during and immediately after the court hearings on 10–11 March 1995 and after the lifting of the ban on revealing Child B's identity on 25 October. News programmes screened at various times throughout the day on the same channel were broadly similar, often using the same film clips and interviews. ITN and Channel 4 news items were similar because ITN supplies news to Channel 4. A *Newsnight* programme on 10 March 1995 included interviews with a consultant specialising in leukaemia and the chief executive of his hospital, a health policy expert, and an expert in medical ethics and law. It also featured a discussion of the case between Stephen Thornton (the health authority chief executive), a leukaemia survivor, and the chief executive of an NHS trust. The *Panorama* programme about the case which was transmitted on 26 October 1995 became a source for many newspaper articles and arguably played a crucial role in promoting Child B to celebrity status.

Early BBC news coverage of the case emphasised the difficult and emotive nature of the issues surrounding it. The opinions of various NHS consultants that the treatment was not warranted because it had only a small chance of success and was likely to be distressing were given some emphasis, and the possibility of treatment doing more harm than good was raised on several occasions by Polly Toynbee and by Cliff Bailey of the UK Children's

Cancer Study Group. Other than Peter Gravett, no doctors were reported in the early period of coverage as arguing that further treatment was appropriate for Child B. On a *Newsnight* programme a survivor of childhood leukaemia was in favour of her being given the treatment, arguing that from a patient's perspective unpleasant treatment was worth putting up with for a chance of life.

Although Cambridge Health Authority was not accused on BBC news programmes of having made its decision on financial grounds alone, the issue of rationing was raised frequently in connection with the case. It was generally presented as something that was inevitable, with discussion focusing on who should make decisions and how. Professor Chris Ham argued that national guideliness were needed, and the chairman of an NHS trust argued that rationing should be done while people are well rather than when they become sick.

BBC coverage in the later period included slightly more criticism of the health authority's decision. On 25 October 1995 a presenter stated that Jaymee was in remission "thanks to private medicine" and that she owed her life to her father and a private benefactor. The following day the *Nine O'Clock News* included criticism of the health authority from Professor John Goldman of the Hammersmith Hospital, who said the decision was too dogmatic and that a compromise should have been reached so she could have been treated. The same news item also included criticism from the Cancer Research Campaign of the government's handling of the case and of the low priority given to research in the NHS.

ITV and Channel 4 also included interviewees who pointed out the difficulties of the decision about whether or not to treat Child B and several times allowed people to say that clinical considerations, rather than financial ones, had dominated the decision. *Channel 4 News* did interview a doctor (Jonathon Waxman, Hammersmith Hospital) who thought that treatment was the best option for Child B and went as far as suggesting that the health authority would be legitimating euthanasia if they did not provide it. His views were partly countered in the same news programme by Richard Nicholson, of the *Bulletin of Medical Ethics*, who questioned whether the treatment was in the child's best interests, noted that the value of bone marrow transplants in leukaemia was now being questioned, and argued that decisions should not be left to doctors who want to try everything possible for an individual patient regardless of costs.

Television coverage of the Child B case did touch on quite a few of the issues it raised and included brief interviews with people able to comment on the case from various perspectives. The comments made by most interviewees, however, were inevitably brief, and debate of the issues on television was thus limited.

Women's magazines

Of 10 high circulation women's magazines contacted, three had covered the case of Child B in one way or another. *Best* magazine had printed a feature article on the case in late September, but it identified Child B as Jaymee Bowen before the ban on identifying her had been lifted and was ordered to retrieve all unsold copies (an event which itself attracted the attention of the *Guardian* newspaper). Although the *Best* feature was not published again, even when the ban had been lifted, the fact that this magazine had the story apparently deterred other women's magazines from covering it. *Hello!* published an interview with Child B's father on 4 November 1995,[80] and *Woman's Own* named Jaymee Bowen as one of its children of courage in the Christmas issue.[81]

In an interview with *Hello!* David Bowen "talk[ed] about his battle to ensure continuing treatment for leukaemia for his young daughter". *Hello!* set out to tell the human side of her story:

> "For months the nation knew her only by a bare brusque initial. She was Child B—a young girl so desperately ill with leukaemia that back in January she was given just eight weeks to live. But now the anonymity order protecting the identity of dark doe-eyed Jaymee Bowen, 11, has been lifted and it's time to tell her human story—a story that has been rather lost among court transcripts, medical statistics and the wider debate on the rationing of NHS treatment".

The article, presented as a series of questions and answers, essentially described Bowen's view of what happened from the time Jaymee's illness recurred in January 1995 to the time of the interview. No comments from elsewhere were included. We quote the description of what motivated him to fight to get further chemotherapy and a second bone transplant in some detail here because it illustrates:

- The strength of his feeling that it was inappropriate to do nothing while there was something that could possibly be done

- His belief that Jaymee was not typical of the children on whom the NHS doctors based their advice because she generally tolerated chemotherapy well
- A point not made elsewhere in the newspaper coverage which condemned the fact that the health authority's decision had been a financial one, that Jaymee's father said he would have understood if the health authority had told him originally that they couldn't afford the treatment.

"When you see your child deteriorating and know that if you do nothing there's a 100 per cent certainty that she will die, there's nothing you can do except push her case a bit further. The hope of finding someone who could help her became, I suppose, like the Star to the Three Wise Men. You are transfixed by the determination to press on".

[Hello! interviewer] You hit the telephone every night for two weeks after the girls were in bed, scouring the country for experts in secondary bone marrow transplants.
"Through the past ten months I've rarely slept more than three or four hours a night... The phone bill came to thousands of pounds, but I didn't give a damn. All the time I was conscious of time running out, but I eventually found two top men in Los Angeles who said she had a 60 per cent chance of surviving the secondary transplant and a 30 per cent chance of being cured. Jaymee was seen by the Hammersmith Hospital consultant I was told was probably the best in the country to carry out the transplant. But then we lost the bed he was holding for her".

You clearly had a very different opinion from Jaymee's original doctors.
"I couldn't understand why Jaymee couldn't be referred or how it could ever be in a child's best interest to die rather than grasp a good chance of living. I couldn't accept the blanket policy to deny children second bone marrow transplants when adult patients were offered the choice... I was told by a doctor that I would be doing my daughter more favours by spending what time she had left with her instead of persisting with my argument".

There was grave concern about the highly toxic chemotherapy that Jaymee faced.
"That was difficult because the chemo can kill you as it's designed to kill all the fastest growing cancer cells in your body. But Jaymee has always reacted to it at once without any problems. Perversely, she only ever got sick from the anti-sickness drug, which we discontinued".

You began your highly stressful legal action because the health authority had said initially that further treatment was not in Jaymee's interest. But later

> *they said they hadn't the funds—£75 000 was needed—for the treatment suggested by Dr Gravett.*
>
> "That was a complete shift of argument—and very hard to bear. If at the start of the eight weeks they'd given Jaymee they had said 'Look, we couldn't afford it', I might not have been happy, but I would have understood. And then I could have used the time fund raising for private treatment. I would have sold my shoes, I would have danced in the street if necessary. But they didn't give me that chance, which was sad".

Woman's Own did not cover the story at the time of the court hearings in March or when the ban on identification was lifted in October. It awarded Jaymee Bowen one of its "Children of Courage" awards, however, and included a profile of her in its Christmas issue. The article started:

> "Last January, in a case that hit the headlines, the health service gave up on Jaymee Bowen. After five years of treatment for leukaemia, they thought they could do no more and gave her just eight weeks to live. But then a mystery benefactor paid for some experimental treatment, and the nation held its breath, praying the 11 year old from Hertfordshire would survive".

It then, as would be expected given that it was focusing on children of courage, described Jaymee's determination and positive attitude. Jaymee's health was said to be currently good, although she was said to be aware that "the odds are stacked against her making a full recovery", and she was described as "a typical 11 year old" at school. The various debates about her treatment were not mentioned nor was the fact that the health authority had refused to pay for the treatment her father wanted and that there had been legal battles, etc.

Health Service Journal

The *Health Service Journal* is a weekly publication containing news, feature, and opinion articles which is targeted primarily at health service managers. Between March 1995 and December 1995 it carried 15 articles primarily about the Child B case and several others that alluded to it. The *Health Service Journal* focused on the wider issues which the case raised, and reports of Child B's personal progress were brief—certainly far less detailed than those appearing in national newspapers at the time.

An editorial article published the week after the first court hearings recognised that the Child B case had "thrust rationing back into public awareness", and predicted that while previous cases of explicit rationing had each "been greeted afresh with public shock and indignation ... this one has highlighted the issues so starkly and unforgettably that it will be a turning point".[82] Certainly within the *Health Service Journal* the Child B case served as a trigger and a focus for wider debate about health care rationing over subsequent months. It is also interesting to note that articles about the case were all listed under the heading "rationing" in the journal's annual index and comprised most of the 20 entries under this heading in 1995. Only 10 articles were indexed under the same heading in 1994.

The editorial article on the Child B case recognised the tension between personal and social values in rationing decisions and asked:

> "What responsible NHS manager could quibble with Cambridge and Huntingdon's decision that, given the child's prognosis, the trauma involved and uncertain outcome, it was only moral to deploy its limited resources elsewhere? Yet what parent would act differently, told their child might have up to a 20% chance of survival?"[82]

The *Health Service Journal* continued to recognise the different viewpoints in the case and juxtaposed Jaymee Bowen's claim that if she met Stephen Thornton she would go over and whack him one with Noel Flannery's praising of Stephen Thornton's integrity and professionalism.

The *Health Service Journal* also argued that a clear, national policy was needed to guide the allocation of resources to individual cases and identified several questions that challenged the "fundamental legitimacy" of health authorities to make appropriate rationing decisions:

> "What scope have their local populations for influencing and challenging their decisions? Are they sure they know the true costs of the treatments they must ration? If not, how can they justify their decisions? What have they done to eradicate ineffective or harmful treatments? ... [Do] they know how their consultants spend every working hour[?][82]

These themes were returned to, with reference to the Child B case, throughout the year.

Although the *Health Service Journal* emphasised in several news reports that Philip Hunt, director of NAHAT (National Association of Health Authorities and Trusts), Noel Flannery, deputy director of IHSM (Institute of Health Service Management), and other senior managers within the health service had praised Cambridge and Huntingdon's handling of the case, it also printed criticisms of the decision. In August space was given to a group of doctors and managers who "offered to prove publicly how the health commission which denied further treatment to a girl dying of leukaemia is wasting resources".[83 84] Ron Zimmern, director of health policy and public health at the commission, countered their criticisms in an Open Space article the following week.[85] In late November, a picture of Jaymee Bowen appeared on the front cover of the journal, which carried a full length article, "Every manager's nightmare" considering what health service managers could learn from the Child B case.[86] This was also quite critical of some aspects of the way Cambridge and Huntingdon Health Commission handled the case and stimulated further correspondence in the journal.

Child B was mentioned in several *Health Service Journal* headlines and articles which were generally about rationing but which did not explore her specific case in any detail. For example, Cambridge and Huntingdon Health Commission was identified as the "Child B" health authority, and several articles were then devoted to a report it produced on health care rationing[87] and criticisms of that report.[83] It seemed that her case both stimulated debate about health care rationing in the *Health Service Journal* and sustained interest in that debate.

British Medical Journal

The *British Medical Journal* is a weekly publication containing original research reports and articles about clinical practice as well as news reports and opinion pieces of particular relevance to medical and related professionals. It published a relatively long news article by its legal correspondent which outlined the main features of the case and the two court judgments.[88] The Child B case and the case of a man with a severe head injury who was flown 320 km by helicopter because local specialist units had no available beds stimulated an editorial in the same issue which argued for a public debate about health care rationing.[89] The editorial noted that Britain has had "a series of brief, heated, and often uninformed debates about particular episodes" but not "the broad, deep, informed, and prolonged debate on rationing that is needed". It pondered whether the latest cases would prompt the necessary debate but thought that debate was likely to die down because the government was unwilling to be candid on rationing.

In early November, an article in the journal's Medicine and the Media section commented on the *Panorama* programme transmitted the week previously and on associated newspaper coverage.[90] Although it concluded that "the media in general behaved rationally in dealing with this difficult issue", the article emphasised that the newspapers failed to deal with the real financial and human costs. Thus, for example,

> "The *Independent* gave one in 40 as Jaymee's initial chances of survival and the cost of treatment so far as about £100 000. This sum may not be much—when there is only one payment and a child is certain to live; the real financial cost per life saved is £4 m".
>
> "Many papers described the treatment as distressing for Jaymee, but none counted the real human cost—that some children with Jaymee's condition would die sooner and with more distress if treated".

The article argued that irrational emotion from Jaymee's father was understandable and that Stephen Thornton and Ross Pinkerton (a leukaemia specialist involved in the original decision) handled difficult questions well on the *Panorama* programme. The author wondered what angle the media would have adopted if Jaymee had died an unpleasant death and her sister had developed complications during donor procedures.

Summary

In this chapter we have outlined some of the key features of media coverage of the Child B case between March and December 1995, focussing particularly on the way the decisions about Child B's treatment were presented. The sheer volume of reporting was striking. The case attracted much prominent coverage in the lay media and was also given a fair amount of attention by relevant specialist media outlets. Child B, even before she was identified, was given celebrity status by the media.

The media varied quite dramatically at times in the way they presented the case, presenting some quite different constructions of what was involved. Generally speaking, beyond consideration of Child B's personal progress, attention was largely focused on the issue of health care rationing. The complex question of whether the treatment was effective, appropriate for Child B, and in her best interests was, after brief consideration at the time of the initial court hearings, largely neglected. The implications of the media coverage of the case, and of the case itself, are discussed further in the next section.

1 Negrine R. *Politics and the mass media in Britain.* London: Routledge, 1989.
2 Anon. Condemned by bank balance. *Sun* 1995 March 11:6.
3 Anon. A price too high to pay. *Daily Mirror* 1995 March 11:6.
4 Anon. Sick system that cheats our children. *Daily Mirror* 1995 March 13:6.
5 Anon. Put a child's life before NHS waste. *Mail on Sunday* 1995 March 12:28.
6 Anon. Questions of life and death. *Daily Mail* 1995 March 11:8.
7 Anon. Weighing health costs. *Daily Telegraph* 1995 March 13:20.
8 Anon. Care in the courts. *Times* 1995 March 11:17.
9 Anon. Open the ration book on health. *Guardian* 1995 March 11:24.
10 Anon. Prayers for the dying. *Daily Express* 1995 March 11:8.
11 Anon. Hard choices: but who decides? *Independent* 1995 March 11:14.
12 Anon. When life costs too much. *Independent on Sunday* 1995 March 12:26.
13 Anon. Shame on you Ginny. *News of the World* 1995 March 12:6.
14 Anon. Trust the patients, not the market. *Observer* 1995 March 12:26.
15 Anon. Jaymee's lesson to us all. *Daily Mirror* 1995 October 26:6.
16 Anon. The limits of the NHS: the question is not whether to ration but how. *Guardian* 1995 October 27:20.
17 Anon. What a girl. *Sun* 1995 October 26:6.
18 Anon. Public waste and a child's will to live. *Daily Mail* 1995 October 26:8.
19 Harrison T. What price a child's life? *Daily Mail* 1995 March 10:1–2.
20 Hope J. How cruel twists of fate shaped a life on borrowed time. *Daily Mail* 1995 March 11:6.
21 Weale S. Dying girl is denied treatment. *Guardian* 1995 March 10:1.
22 Anon. A five year fight for survival . . . the story of little "B". *Daily Mirror* 1995 March 11:5.
23 Davies C, Holden W. Hope then crushing defeat, all in the space of six hours. *Daily Telegraph* 1995 March 11:4.
24 Anon. NHS rethink on Child B. *Guardian* 1995 August 23:8.
25 Midgley C. Daily Mirror offers to pay for dying girl's op. *Daily Mirror* 1995 March 11:1–2.
26 Anon. Her health in their hands. *Daily Mirror* 1995 March 11:5.
27 Anon. The pool party pooper. *Daily Mirror* 1995 October 26:5.
28 Midgley C. Second class, doc: casual letter to seal the fate of tragic cancer girl B. *Daily Mirror* 1995 March 13:4–5.
29 Mullin J. Father sees hope for leukaemia girl vanish in volte-face. *Guardian* 1995 March 11:5.
30 Mihill C. Leukaemia girl warned of 1pc chance. *Guardian* 1995 March 14:2.
31 Laurance J. NHS specialists advised against second operation: the treatment. *Times* 1995 March 11:3.
32 Toynbee P. Did the NHS cheat Jaymee? *Independent* 1995 October 27:23.

33 Brindle D. MPs call for firmer NHS treatment rules. *Guardian* 1995 March 13:5.
34 Stuttaford T. Success of earlier treatment makes for poor prognosis. *Times* 1995 March 13:3.
35 Hall C. Leukaemia success story hides agony of luckless minority. *Independent* 1995 March 11:3.
36 O'Connor AM. Effects of framing and level of probability on patients' preference for cancer chemotherapy. *J Clin Epidemiol* 1989;**42**:119–26.
37 Dunn J. This bed is ready NOW. Just give me the chance to save her. *Daily Mirror* 1995 March 11:2–3.
38 Davies C. Let's get on with it, says leukaemia girl. *Daily Telegraph* 1995 March 14:8.
39 Davies C, Jones G. Leukaemia girl responds well to first drugs. *Daily Telegraph* 1995 March 15:10.
40 Anon. Cancer girl treated. *Guardian* 1995 March 15:2.
41 Laurance C. Girl "B" begins cancer therapy. *Times* 1995 March 15:2.
42 Reade B, Midgley C. Teddy in one hand, tv zapper in the other, B declares: I feel fine. *Daily Mirror* 1995 March 15:9.
43 Wood M. Plucky miss B's full of beans! *Sun* 1995 March 15:10.
44 Marks K. Judge will rule today on girl's right to life. *Daily Telegraph* 1995 March 10:5.
45 Hall C. Policy issues cloud decisions over treatment. *Independent* 1995 March 11:3.
46 Anon. Court judges lawfulness of decision: law report. *Times* 1995 March 15: 23.
47 Jones J. Should we save only the young? *Observer* 1995 October 29:20.
48 Anon. Father who beat all the odds. *Sunday Express* 1995 March 12:11.
49 Palmer J. Final hurdle for cancer experts. *Daily Mirror* 1995 March 13:4.
50 Paxton C. Letters. *Times* 1995 March 20:17.
51 Le Fanu J. Who'll have the last word? *Daily Telegraph* 1995 March 11:23.
52 Anon. They spend £225 million a year on AIDS. Why can't the NHS find £75,000 for a child with cancer? *Sunday Express* 1995 March 12:10–11.
53 Fenton B. Leukaemia girl faces heavy chemotherapy. *Daily Telegraph* 1995 March 13:2.
54 Collee J. Dr John Collee on the dangers of media appeals to save sick children's lives. *Observer (Life)* 1995 July 2:62.
55 Allen D. Did they let our little girl die too? *News of the World* 1995 March 12: 20–21.
56 Anon. Public interest grounds necessary: law report. *Times* 1995 March 15:23.
57 Reade B, Midgley C. My B heard her own story on radio news and said to me: she must have the op, dad. *Daily Mirror* 1995 March 13:1.
58 Anon. Girl B "eager for treatment". *Times* 1995 March 14:1.
59 Pukas A. The right to live? *Sunday Times* 1995 March 12:16.
60 Pierce A. Family of leukaemia girl prepares her for last chance of life. *Times* 1995 March 13:3.
61 Penman D. Family urged to tell leukaemia girl the truth. *Independent* 1995 March 13:7.
62 Rice D. I'll treat your girl, but you must tell her she's dying. *Sunday Mirror* 1995 March 124–5.
63 Midgley C. I'm not scared Daddy. *Daily Mirror* 1995 March 14:1.
64 Kay J. I'll start treatment to save little B's life today. *Sun* 1995 March 13:4.
65 Howard M. My son's ill—but I disagree with B's dad. *Sunday Mirror* 1995 March 12:4–5.
66 Harrison T. The injection of hope: pioneering treatment for cancer girl refused cash. *Daily Mail* 1995 April 5:16.

67 Duce R. Experimental therapy for Child B. *Times* 1995 April 5:5.
68 Mihill C. Leukaemia girl's "guinea pig" hope. *Guardian* 1995 April 5:7.
69 Midgley C. My "B" is guinea pig ... but every day's precious. *Daily Mirror* 1995 April 5:11.
70 Anon. It works miracles ... but no-one knows how. *Daily Express* 1995 April 5:17.
71 Fowler R. Courage of an 11 year old's battle for life. *Independent* 1995 October 26:3.
72 Paxton A, Frost B. Hope for Girl B after survival of boy "not worth treating". *Times* 1995 March 20:1.
73 Davis C. Sacrificing my chance of survival wasn't easy. *Daily Telegraph* 1995 March 15:10.
74 Doyle C. Moral dilemma as NHS adds up cost of living. *Daily Telegraph* 1995 March 11:5.
75 Anon. Message of hope. *Daily Mirror* 1995 March 11:2.
76 Mihill C. Guideline plea for rationing of treatment. *Guardian* 1995 March 11: 5.
77 O'Grady J. How can you hang a price tag on a human life? *Daily Telegraph* 1995 October 26:18.
78 Brindle D. Secret summit plans rationing for NHS: top doctors told priority setting is "inevitable". *Guardian* 1995 October 27:1–2.
79 d'Ancona M. How child B fought cancer with courage. *Times* 1995 October 28:20.
80 Kingsley M. Jaymee Bowen "Child B". *Hello!* 1995 November 4:66–70.
81 Anon. Britain's bravest little fighters. *Woman's Own* 1995 December 18/25: 74–7.
82 Anon. Rationing needs a rational policy. *Health Service Journal* 1995 March 16: 17.
83 Chadda D. Anti-rationing group issues public challenge to "Child B" authority. *Health Service Journal* 1995 August 17:5.
84 Crosby D, Dunn R, Evans K, Grundy P, Hopkins R, Lewis P, *et al.* Allow us to test the wisdom of rationing. *Health Service Journal* 1995 August 17:16.
85 Zimmern R. Insufficient to simply be efficient. *Health Service Journal* 1995 August 24:19.
86 Wall A. Every manager's mightmare. *Health Service Journal* 1995 November 30:24–6.
87 Anon. Rationing report from "Child B" HA. *Health Service Journal* 1995 June 1:6.
88 Dyer C. Girl with leukaemia will be treated privately. *BMJ* 1995;**310**:687.
89 Smith R. Rationing: the debate we have to have. *BMJ* 1995;**310**:686.
90 Goodman NW. Child B is revealed. *BMJ* 1995;**311**:1235.

What are the implications of the Child B case for the debate on health care policies?

IAN S WATT, VIKKI A ENTWISTLE

In the first part of this chapter we described how the media covered the Child B case from March to December 1995. Now we discuss some of the issues raised by the media coverage and by the case itself. We consider the following themes: the basis of decisions about treatment (clinical and financial considerations); the allocation of public funds; the expectation that something can and should be done to save every ill child; health technology assessment and considerations of health care effectiveness; the concept of informed patient choice in health care; the role of medical advice; the portrayal of doctors and health service managers; and the selection of commentators. We conclude by considering how well the media performed and what role(s) they fulfilled in their coverage of the Child B case.

Studies of media content, such as that reported in the previous section, cannot tell us with any degree of certainty about the flows of information and production processes underlying it (how the content came to be the way it was), how well it reflected what actually happened, or how people understood, interpreted, and used it. Although media texts can provide some clues as to their origins, they tend to obscure a variety of interactions between information sources, journalists, and their editors. Among audiences, people may derive different meanings from the same media texts, and their understanding may not be that which was intended by journalists or programme producers. For example, Caroline van den Brul found that four out of twelve people who had left school at 16 misunderstood television news clips reporting the possibility that vitamin K injections given to babies might cause childhood leukaemia. Three of them thought that vitamin K injections were given to prevent leukaemia.[1] In the absence of empirical research on the subject we can only speculate about how people understood media coverage of the Child B case and about the impact it had.

Perceptions of the characters and issues involved in the Child B case are likely to be affected by knowledge of her current health status. Judgments about the correctness or otherwise of the decisions by NHS consultants not to provide further treatment for Child B, by her father and Dr Gravett to go ahead with treatment, and by the health authority not to fund it will inevitably be influenced by knowledge of the outcome of those decisions. While we were conducting our study of media coverage of the case up until December 1995, Child B was in remission and apparently relatively healthy. She died, however, in May 1996.

The basis of treatment decisions: clinical and financial considerations

Large sections of the media, particularly the tabloid press, presented the Child B case as an example of the rationing of care within the NHS. Child B was introduced in news reports as the girl with leukaemia who was denied expensive treatment by the NHS. While it is certainly true that the issue of resources was considered once the case was in the courts, the doctors who initially advised against further treatment may have done so for purely clinical reasons, believing that it was not in Child B's best interests to receive treatments with serious adverse side effects when they offered very little prospect of improvement in prognosis. A study of the *All England Law Report* on the Appeal Court decision found that in the Child B case there was "no evidence to show that the doctor was modifying her clinical judgment with considerations about resources".[2] Thus, although the case was widely heralded as an example of health care rationing, it is possible to argue that essentially it was no such thing.

Once Child B's father approached the health authority to ask them to fund the treatment the issue of resources had to play a part in the decision because the health authority, as it argued in the Appeal Court, had to bear in mind its responsibility to a wider community and consider the opportunity costs of treatment. As Price pointed out, the rational structure of the question of whether or not to treat Child B seems to have changed when the case was taken to the health authority (or at least when it reached the courts). "It ceased to be about B's best interests and about responding to suffering, and became instead an issue of costs, benefits and resource availability".[2] There was an apparent switch from an argument about what was in the best interests of an individual child to a broadly utilitarian argument about what was in the best interests of a wider community.

In connection with the Child B case all the national news media studied raised questions about the allocation of resources within the NHS. Some framed the question of whether scarce resources should be used to give Child B the treatment her father wanted in terms of what greater benefits could be gained if it was spent otherwise (for example, on more effective treatments for other patients), while others framed it in terms of how much more benefit would be gained by spending it on Child B than on other less gainful or less worthy causes (for example, on cosmetic surgery or abortions). It is interesting to note that while various sectors of the media quite confidently introduced the concept of opportunity cost into their coverage of the case, they did not discuss the limitations of the cost-effectiveness data which might inform rationing decisions and the value judgments which would inevitably be introduced in decisions about which treatments should be provided to which people and which should not.

Although the media provided several examples of what £75 000 could buy if it was not spent on further chemotherapy and a second bone marrow transplant for Child B, they either did not attempt to or, if they did attempt to would have found it very difficult to, disentangle and identify precisely who among the population of Cambridge and Huntingdon received health care bought with that money. This is perhaps a good thing; the prospect of trials by media of the merits and deserts of those patients who benefited from a particular opportunity cost foregone is not appealing.

Neither the nature and status of evidence about the effectiveness of further aggressive chemotherapy and a second bone marrow transplant in relapsed cases of acute myeloid leukaemia nor the likelihood of Child B surviving were particularly clearly presented in media accounts. Media reports presented various estimates of the chances of Child B surviving (or at least going into remission) with treatment, although the uncertainty underlying these was not emphasised. The inclusion of these estimates meant that the issue was framed so that the likely downsides of treatment had to be valued relative to the (small, but positive) chances of survival. Although it was often emphasised that Child B would certainly die without further treatment, it was never clearly stated that there had been no instances in which children with relapsed acute myeloid leukaemia had survived, with or without treatment. Several children who had survived despite being given gloomy prognoses were presented in the media, usually together with messages from their parents or themselves that it was worth opting for treatment but they had apparently not relapsed like Child B. If it had been made clear that there had been no such instances of children with relapsed acute myeloid leukaemia recovering, this may have led people to think that nothing short of a miracle would save Child B and that the unpleasantness of the proposed treatment and its likely side effects would almost certainly be in vain. The context for interpretation, however, was otherwise set. The failure of many media reports to distinguish between permanent cure and temporary remission when they mentioned chances of success of treatment is also likely to have influenced interpretations of the various judgments about whether further treatment was appropriate.

The question of whether the decision not to fund treatment for Child B was based on consideration of the child's best interests or the interests of wider society and whether it was made on grounds of effectiveness of cost-effectiveness was rarely covered in the media. There are several possible reasons for the fact that newspapers seemed either to start from the assumption that it was a case of health care rationing or to lose sight of the clinical considerations in the case. For example, some journalists may not have been aware of the strength and consensus of the views of the NHS consultants treating Child B, possibly because the viewpoints of those fighting for further treatment were more actively and persuasively given to them than the viewpoints of those opposed to further treatment, and possibly because the courts focused heavily on the issues of resource allocation. Journalists might have been tempted to play down the clinical arguments against treating her because the rationing angle made for a "stronger" story (the denial of "necessary" treatment to a child being more newsworthy than the reluctance to provide a treatment which may cause harm). The balance of the reporting may also have been affected by reluctance among doctors closely concerned with the case to speak publicly about Child B's personal clinical details because this would break confidentiality. Doctors not familiar with the case may have been reluctant to comment on it.

We have to consider the fact that the NHS, whether we like it or not, is now regularly viewed in a political light. This may mean that even decisions which are primarily about clinical effectiveness and a patient's best interests tend to be *seen* as examples of health care rationing. The language currently used to discuss health care issues within the market oriented NHS may exacerbate this tendency. An article in the *Independent on Sunday* pointed out that treatments are now "funded" rather than "provided" and argued quite persuasively that if people are told about treatment decisions in a language which has been developed from a basis in economics rather than compassion, they will quite naturally think that money has dominated those decisions.[3]

The argument that resource issues should be kept out of individual doctor–patient relationships and should be introduced into decision making only at a managerial level is, at least superficially, appealing. In a cash limited system, however, it could lead to unpleasant situations in which clinical decisions made by doctors (or doctors and patients) were "overruled" and patients were denied treatments which they had been led to believe they could have. It may not be possible (and may not necessarily be desirable) for clinical decisions to be made completely devoid of cost considerations. Even if costs are not explicitly taken into account, economic factors may subconsciously or indirectly influence clinical decision making. Whatever happened in the Child B case we know that, as several media reports acknowledged, resources and costs have been borne in mind by doctors making decisions about individual patients in their care. For example, doctors have had to decide which people with end stage kidney disease would benefit from renal dialysis technology because there simply were not enough facilities to allow all those who might have benefited from it to do so. While many doctors in the United Kingdom fail to recognise their rationing decisions this is not the case in many other countries. The gross imbalance between need and resources in parts of the developing world means that doctors' implicit rationing is more readily recognised.

The allocation of public funds

In reporting that was directly connected with the case there were a few instances in which journalists or others questioned whether it would still be necessary to ration state-provided health care if more public funds were diverted to health care from other expenditures or if taxes were raised. Outside of the Child B case the media regularly present news items and features which highlight a number of ways in which resources are spent on things other than health care. They bring to people's attention, for example, spending on defence, the arts, and glamorous lifestyles for a small minority. The media may thus provoke consideration of public spending priorities across society and not just within the health service. By providing a view of the opportunity costs of public spending outside the NHS the media may tend to make it harder for people to accept curtailment of health care which they perceive they or others need.

The expectation that something can, should, and will be done

Media coverage of the Child B case might be seen as an indicator of a widespread expectation that modern medicine can cure every ill and provide a solution to every problem. In particular, much of the news reporting of this case was consistent with the expectation that there is nearly always something which can and should be done to prevent a child from dying. While some more reflective pieces commented on the difficulties which people today have in accepting that children sometimes die, the point remains that expectations may sometimes be unrealistic.

Much, although not all, media coverage expressed sympathy for the feeling that all possible medical technologies should be tried, particularly when a life is at stake. It also reflected the view that, at least in "deserving" cases, they should be provided by the NHS. When the NHS "failed" to provide these technologies the media accepted with little comment that people would seek them privately and would do what they could to raise the money to do so.

Health technology assessment and issues of effectiveness

The issue of clinical effectiveness is currently high on the NHS agenda. It is increasingly recognised that clinical practice should reflect research evidence about the effectiveness of interventions and that new technologies should be evaluated and be shown to be effective before they are widely introduced. Some media reports did make a distinction between treatment which is known to be effective and that which is of unproved benefit, although some confusion may have arisen about the status of the treatments proposed for Child B because small probabilities of success were often quoted as if they were definite and correct.

Reporting of the Child B case probably conveyed an accurate impression that at least some developments in modern medicine occur in a fairly haphazard way. It was unlikely, however, to inform people about current standards for health technology assessment and how we come to reliable knowledge of whether treatments are effective. For example, the difference between observing what happens to one child who is given an "experimental" treatment and carrying out a rigorous evaluation with an appropriate experimental design was rarely even alluded to. The limitations of the estimates of the chances of treatment being successful were rarely discussed, and the difficulties of generalising from research reports of the average effects of interventions among particular groups to individual cases was not well explored.

Several media reports incorporated comments to the effect that if people were not willing to see new treatments tried on people like Child B no more progress could be made in medicine. The more subtle point that reliable advances in knowledge could arise only if new treatments were tried within the context of a rigorous trial was less frequently made. There may have been an implicit assumption underlying some of the media coverage of this case that a new treatment would necessarily be better than existing ones. The point that the possible harms of new, unevaluated treatments may be greater than those of existing treatments was not fully explored (although the appropriateness of certain last chance, high technology treatments for dying children was occasionally questioned in the early stages of the case). It is not clear to what extent media coverage of this case would have helped people understand the limited nature of available research evidence about the effectiveness of health care interventions, or about the inherent uncertainty attached to medical decision making.

The conduct and use of effectiveness research in public and private health care sectors

In Britain, research to evaluate health care effectiveness takes place largely within NHS settings, even when it is funded from commercial rather than governmental or charitable sources. Clinical effectiveness is arguably a more pressing concern for publicly funded health systems than for private sector health care providers (although medical insurance companies obviously have concerns about effectiveness and even cost-effectiveness too). As long as people are willing to pay, the private sector can afford to focus on individual perceptions of need and effectiveness. The public sector needs to take a broader view, in which population as well as individual needs and outcome data, cost-effectiveness as well as effectiveness data, are important.

If decisions about treatment taken in the private sector are less likely to be influenced by considerations of effectiveness and cost-effectiveness, the private sector may be more likely to provide less effective or even harmful treatments than the NHS (in addition, of course, to providing effective but very expensive treatments). Of course, if the private sector was to gain a reputation among potential patients for providing ineffective treatments or causing harm this situation could change.

Much media coverage of the Child B case presented the private sector in a neutral light. The facts that Child B had been admitted to a private hospital and that Dr Gravett was a Harley Street consultant were almost always introduced without explicit comment about the relative merits of the private sector and the NHS or of Harley Street consultants as compared with any other consultants. Obviously the varying constructions of the story may have tended to influence perceptions. A few articles did explicitly emphasise that private sector health care was giving Child B a chance of life which the NHS had not, but there were no explicit suggestions that the private sector was sanctioning an intervention which was more likely to do harm than good.

Informed patient choice

NHS policy currently promotes the greater involvement of patients in decisions about their care. This reflects an underlying tendency for paternalistic approaches in health care to fall from favour while consumerist approaches are increasingly seen as acceptable. Shared decision making, in which health professionals and patients discuss options and agree on a course of action, is generally seen as the most desirable model.

The Patient's Charter has stated since 1991 that patients have a right to "be given a clear explanation of any treatment proposed, including any risks and any alternatives, before you decide whether you will agree to the treatment".[4] One of the current priority objectives for the NHS is that "purchasers and providers should be able to demonstrate that they have a systematic programme in place aimed at achieving active partnership with individual patients in their own care, in particular seeking to improve the quantity and quality of information given to enable patient choice about treatment options".[5]

When Child B relapsed in January 1995 the consultant responsible for her care and the consultant from whom a second opinion was sought both advised against (and, it seems, refused to carry out) further aggressive treatment. Child B's father did not accept this advice so he and the doctors were unable to reach a mutually acceptable shared decision. This, and the difficulties which may be more generally experienced with attempts to implement shared decision making, were rarely explored in coverage of the case.

If we assume that the doctors' advice was based on purely clinical grounds and that they believed they were acting in the child's best interests then their approach may be characterised as paternalistic. In so far as Child B's father had decided what treatment he wanted (and later actively sought someone to provide it) his approach quite definitely fitted a consumerist model of health care. The situation is slightly more complex in this case, however, because the patient was a child. Her father might also be described as having taken a paternalistic approach, although he had different ideas about what was in her best interests than the doctors did. (It is possible that the father's opinions about what was best for his daughter were clouded by his own needs).

There is as yet no clear consensus about the extent to which children can or should be involved in treatment decisions, although there have recently been calls for further discussion of the issues and the promotion of more appropriate involvement than is currently the case.[6] Several newspaper articles and television items quoted people who either noted the absence of information about Child B's own preference regarding further treatment or argued that her views should be considered, but the media did not particularly criticise either the doctors or her father for any perceived paternalism on their part. The consumerist approach of Child B's father also attracted little comment as such, although when he announced his intention to sue the health authority for negligence in his daughter's care, the *Observer* did note that this was "not quite the assertive 'patient power' the government had in mind when it launched its Patient's Charter four years ago".[7]

If people are to make informed choices about health care treatments they need to know what the options are and how they compare. If the range of available options differs from the range of possible options (which it is increasingly likely to do in publicly funded health care systems, given limited resources and rapid developments in medical technology) then the question of which options they should be told about arises. Some would argue that people should be told about all possible options so they can decide for themselves whether they want to, and are able and willing to, seek an option which is not readily available to them on the NHS from elsewhere. Health professionals often will not know what financial resources people may be willing to access or what trade offs they may be willing to make between wealth and health. Some people, however, may want to but be unable to access or raise money for private treatments. Those who are aware of and desire treatments which they cannot obtain may experience deprivation disutility. This may have negative consequences, including adverse effects on health, at an individual level. At a social level it may lead to pressure for change with a variety of possible positive or negative effects. The pros and cons of informing people about all possible or only available options may appear differently to people who think within different theoretical or philosophical frameworks in relation to health care provision and the involvement of patients in treatment decisions.[8]

The role of medical advice

Media coverage of the Child B case raised the question of to what extent people should listen to and have confidence in doctors' advice. Readers and viewers saw one man question the doctors who said his daughter was at death's door, fight for treatment that many doctors argued against, and see his daughter survive, at least in the short term. The publicity which the case attracted certainly had the potential to reduce the trust which parents put in medical doctors, both because it could raise awareness of the uncertainty of much medical knowledge and because it could tend to make people suspicious that when doctors advise against treatment they may be motivated by cost considerations rather than by concern to do what is best for the patient. This was starkly illustrated by the father of a child who had died of leukaemia, who questioned whether he had done enough (see p 119).

If people think that the NHS will always tend to undertreat because of resource considerations they may be less convinced that the care they are offered or given is adequate and may be more inclined to seek more treatment (which may not always be likely to secure them more health gain), possibly from the private sector.

Despite the fact that the first (and then apparently most) doctors who considered Child B's case advised against further treatment, media coverage of the case might have raised awareness of the possibility that doctors could be overridden by health authorities in decisions about expensive treatments, whether these treatments were effective or not. The case of a young boy with cystic fibrosis, which was reported in the newspapers alongside the Child B case in several instances, involved a situation in which his doctor had recommended an expensive new drug treatment which the local health authority had refused to fund. Several newspaper and television reports briefly introduced the concept of doctors acting as patients' advocates, fighting on their behalf to secure the required or desired treatments. This role, however, was not fully explored.

The portrayal of doctors and health service managers

To some extent, interpretations of media presentations of the characters involved in the Child B case will always be dependent on knowledge of the outcomes of the treatment she was given. When Child B went into remission in May 1995 it was easy for both journalists and their audiences to assume that the NHS consultants and the health authority had got things awfully wrong and that her father and Dr Gravett were vindicated heroes.

Media coverage tended to paint a fairly negative picture of health service managers, while doctors escaped relatively unscathed. Media reports which acknowledged that doctors have been making rationing decisions implicitly for years did not criticise them for choosing which patients to treat and which not to. Health service managers, who now make similar decisions more openly and are less able than doctors to ignore questions of cost-effectiveness, did not escape so lightly. It is relatively easy for journalists to present health service managers as callous bureaucrats. The image of health authorities in reporting about the Child B case was not improved by the fact that journalists linked shortages of resources for patient care with wastage and excess in health service administration and management.

The general tendency to portray health authorities and the individuals who serve on them in a negative light may have serious consequences for the way rationing issues are discussed in public. If sections of the media continue to scapegoat those who have to make decisions about health care priorities, people may become less willing to be honest about the decisions they face and make (or may even be pressured into not making the decisions they feel they ought). This may drive rationing decisions back into secrecy and is likely to stifle serious consideration and debate about the issues.

The NHS consultants who advised against further treatment for Child B were rarely explicitly criticised in the media. Even the *Daily Mirror*, which so ardently argued that Child B should be given treatment, focused its explicit criticisms on the way they (or the health care system) had told her father that her condition had deteriorated rather than on the quality of their clinical advice. There are several possible reasons for this. Firstly, very few doctors (particularly specialists) would have disagreed with their clinical judgment. The treatment of (and research into) childhood cancers is well coordinated within the United Kingdom, and there is a remarkably high level of agreement among specialists about treatment protocols. Journalists would therefore have found it very hard (as indeed Child B's father did) to find anyone who disagreed and would have found it even harder to find anyone who would disagree publicly. Codes of good practice within medicine outlaw "unnecessary or unsustainable" public criticism of other doctors,[10] and the concept of professional autonomy or clinical freedom makes doctors loath to speak out against the clinical practice of individual colleagues. It is also possible that a general "reverence" for medical skill influenced the media portrayal of the doctors associated with this case. Although it has been argued recently that the media (and television in particular) now present a much more challenging view of medicine and medical practice than was previously the case, coverage still "displays clear ideological support for the medical profession".[11]

Dr Gravett was enthusiastically portrayed as a benevolent hero in some tabloid reports, and his image was boosted once Child B went into remission, returned to school, and enjoyed her 11th birthday party. Broadsheet news coverage was less adulatory but was rarely explicitly critical. Dr Gravett's motives were not questioned, and the possibility that he might, as a private practitioner, gain financially from the case, particularly because of the publicity it attracted, was not explored. Again, professional ethics are likely to have protected him from direct criticism by other doctors. A few more explicitly sceptical broadsheet articles pointed out that Dr Gravett was outside the mainstream of (respected) NHS childhood cancer specialists, and that he was willing to undertake treatments which most orthodox experts would not do.

The selection of authorised commentators

Information and comment relating to the Child B case was attributed to quite a variety of people. At the time of the court case, the arguments put forward by solicitors for both Child B's father and the health authority were widely reported, as were those of judges in the High Court and Appeal Court. Throughout the coverage, several of those most intimately involved in the case were quoted extensively. Their contributions to the "human interest" aspects of the story, building up pictures of Child B's character and life and of the feelings of those around her, were particularly prominent in tabloid journalism but certainly not absent from the more highbrow media outlets. Comments from Child B's father, grandfather, stepmother, and headteacher were all fairly widely reported. Dr Gravett was regularly quoted, particularly once treatment had started and he was obviously the person most eligible to supply "progress reports".

The NHS consultants who advised against further treatment for Child B did not make any public comments until Ross Pinkerton appeared in the *Panorama* programme in October 1995. In contrast, the health authority's chief executive, Stephen Thornton, featured quite regularly in newspaper and television reports throughout the case, rehearsing a consistent message about what underlay the health authority's decision despite very negative portrayals by certain parts of the media.

Most people who were not directly connected with the case but who were given a voice in media reports were, apart from the journalists and columnists themselves, specialist medical professionals (supplying background information about leukaemia and its treatments or observations on some of the more clinical issues raised by the case) or senior figures in health service management (generally talking about how treatment and funding decisions are made and about rationing in health care). A few politicians, including the then secretary of state of health, Virginia Bottomley, also featured. It is interesting to reflect on the types of people and groups whose viewpoints did not feature. These include Child B's mother, churches and other religious groups, representatives of the NHS research and development programme, general practitioners, and public health specialists. Although a few individual members of the wider public were given space to comment on letters pages, there were few obvious attempts by the media to elicit and report the views of the public and certainly nothing which could be said to represent an informed public debate.

It is not clear from the analysis of content to what extent the people who did feature in media coverage proactively offered information and comment and to what extent they were responding to requests initiated by journalists. Similarly, it is not clear whether those who did not feature to any great extent (such as the NHS consultants at Addenbrookes and the Royal Marsden hospitals) were not asked for comments or refused to supply them.

The emotional appeal of children

To a large extent, media coverage of the Child B case focused on the fact that a sick child was involved and reflected the view that priority should be given to doing whatever was possible for a child. Public opinion surveys have also suggested that people in the developed industrial world generally think that children should be given preference in situations in which health care may be rationed.[12] The perceived primacy of the child within present society perhaps warrants more critical consideration than it has tended to be given. It is not a universal value, and in some more traditional societies greater value is placed on older people.

A child with cancer is a very emotive cause, highly likely to attract public sympathy and to affect people's perceptions of health care priorities. The emotive appeal of Child B was enhanced by the way the media portrayed her personality and built up her status to that of a major celebrity. Even early coverage of the case, particularly in the *Daily Mirror*, was concerned to show that, despite her anonymity, Child B was a person with a distinctive character rather than a statistic. Reporters spent time with her and newspapers (even the broadsheets, to a certain extent) found space to descibe her personality, her favourite toys, and her likes and dislikes in terms of pop stars and food. The *Panorama* programme, which revealed her face and introduced a mass public audience to a remarkable, spirited child, ensured that more people would feel as though they knew her, would be struck by the fact that so far the contested further treatment seemed to be paying off, and would want to be kept informed about her future progress.

The media and public debate about rationing and other health care issues

The Child B case highlighted dilemmas, tensions, and problems in many aspects of health care and health policy. In its treatment of the story of a child whom it raised to celebrity status it raised practical and ethical questions about the introduction of unproved treatments; the roles of clinicians, patients, and managers in treatment decisions; what should be done when doctors and patients disagree; the impact of the internal market in health care on decision making processes and public perception of health care; health care rationing and the provision of expensive treatments on the NHS; and the relation between the NHS and the private sector.

Media reports about the case touched on many relevant questions and, taken as a whole, covered an impressive range of issues. Anyone who read or dipped into only one newspaper, however, would have received a very limited and partial view of the case and the issues it raised. We should recognise that the media did not set out to provide an in depth analysis of the issues raised by the Child B case and that it is not appropriate to criticise them for failing to do what they did not set out to do. In terms of providing reports which were of widespread interest, sold newspapers, and held the attention of viewers and listeners, media coverage of the Child B case seems to have been highly successful.

There have been many calls recently, including from within different sectors of the media, for a public debate about some of the issues raised by the Child B case and particularly about health care rationing. Specific practical suggestions as to how this debate should happen have been less frequent. While the broadsheet newspapers published some critical letters from readers and the *Daily Mirror* and *Sun* published calls and letters of support for Child B and her family, these did not constitute an informed public debate.

The media did provide information (although it tended to be limited) and opinion (although from a limited range of regular journalists and authorised commentators) about the Child B case in particular and some of the general issues it highlighted. Our study suggests that while the media may raise awareness of the issues which need debating, and may influence people's perceptions of these issues they do not provide the solid base of information which would allow people to participate in debates in a particularly informed way, and their coverage itself does not constitute a full public debate.

1 Van den Brul C. *Perceptions of science: how scientists and others view the media reporting of science*. 6th Guardian Lecture. Oxford: Nuffield College, 1994.
2 Price D. Lessons for health care rationing from the case of child B. *BMJ* 1996; **312**:167–9.
3 Victor P, Penman D. New NHS-speak has no word for compassion: "Girl B"—communication failure. *Independent on Sunday, Britain in Focus*; 12 March 1995: 3.
4 Department of Health. *The patient's charter*. London: HMSO, 1991.
5 NHS Executive. *Priorities and planning guidance, 1996/7*. London: NHS Executive, 1995.
6 Alderson P, Montgomery J. What about me? Are children competent to decide on their own treatment? *Health Service Journal*; 11th April 1996:22–4.
7 Jones J. Should we save only the young? *Independent* 29 October 1996:20.
8 Entwistle VA, Sheldon TA, Sowden AJ, Watt IS. Supporting consumer involvement in decision making: what constitutes quality in consumer health information? *International Journal for Quality in Health Care* 1996: in press.
9 Allen D. Did they let our little angel die too? *News of the World* 12 March 1995: 20–1.
10 General Medical Council (1995). *Good medical practice: guidance from the General Medical Council*. London.
11 Bury M, Gabe J. Television and medicine: medical dominance or trial by media? In: Gabe J, Kelleher D, Williams G (Eds) 1994 *Challenging medicine*. London: Routledge, 65–83.
12 Lewis PA, Charny M. Which of two individuals do you treat when only their ages are different and you can't treat both? *Journal of Medical Ethics* 1989;**15**: 28–32.

Postscript: Media coverage of the death of Child B

VIKKI A ENTWISTLE, IAN S WATT

Jaymee Bowen, Child B, died in the evening of Tuesday 21 May 1996. Her death was widely reported by the broadcast media the following day and by national daily newspapers on Thursday 23 May. Following our previous study of media coverage of the Child B case from March to December 1995, we now report on a content analysis of media coverage immediately after Jaymee Bowen's death, paying particular attention to retrospective views of the case and the issues it raised.

Our media sample comprised the BBC's *Nine O'Clock News*, *Channel 4 News*, and ITN's *News at Ten* of 22 May 1996 and one issue of each of the *Daily Express*, *Daily Mail*, *Daily Mirror*, *Daily Telegraph*, *Guardian*, *Independent*, *Sun*, and *Times* (usually a Scottish edition) dated 23 May 1996. Each programme or newspaper was scanned for items or articles about Child B or explicitly linked to her case. The content of these was then systematically studied, with all mentions of the following themes being recorded: the health authority's decision not to fund the treatment; what the experimental treatment achieved and how that was valued; and what the case was seen as highlighting.

Jaymee Bowen's death was widely and prominently reported, confirming the celebrity status she had achieved during the last 15 months of her life. She was mentioned on the front page of every national newspaper on 23 May and most newspapers included several articles about her case. Table 5.3 shows the number of articles and pictures included in each of the newspapers studied.

The media included numerous tributes to Jaymee Bowen's character. Clips and quotations taken from her appearance on the

Table 5.3 Number of articles of different types, number of pictures (excluding pictures of journalists), and number of pages on which Jaymee Bowen appeared on 23 May 1996

Newspaper	News	Leaders	Features/ comment	Pictures	Pages
Daily Express	2 + banner	0	1	4	3
Daily Mail	1 + banner	0	1	3	4
Daily Mirror	4	1	0	17	6
Daily Telegraph	3	1	3	4	4
Guardian	1	1	0	1	3
Independent	4	0	0	2	2
Sun	7	1	1	12	6
Times	5	0	1	5	4

BBC *Panorama* programme transmitted on 26 October 1995 were widely repeated and used particularly to emphasise her courage and determination. In addition, several print journalists explicitly claimed the privilege of having got to know Jaymee and shared insights into her character and views in fairly lengthy feature articles. We suggest that the huge amount of interest in the case was at least partly due to Jaymee Bowen's strong personality as well, of course, as her willingness to talk with reporters.

Several newspapers emphasised the painless and peaceful nature of Jaymee Bowen's death and the fact that she had a smile on her lips before she died. The coverage was reminiscent of attempts to console grieving relatives about the way a loved one has died. *Channel 4 News* noted that doctors said she had died without discomfort and with her family at her side. While much of the media coverage at the time of her death was personal and emotional, however, there was also a fair amount of retrospective comment on aspects of the Child B case.

Reflections on the health authority's decision not to fund treatment

The national newspapers continued to differ quite dramatically in the way they portrayed Cambridge Health Authority's decision not to fund the further chemotherapy and a second bone marrow transplant, which Child B's father wanted for her but which her doctors advised against. The *Daily Mirror* and more particularly the

Sun, in keeping with their earlier coverage of the case, remained critical of the fact that Child B was not given treatment on the NHS. The *Daily Mirror* editorial declared that Jaymee was an "inspiration for the way she fought leukaemia and the bureaucrats of the health service" and argued that "the health service bureaucrats are concerned only with money, not with caring and human emotions".[1]

The *Sun* editorial described how "her devoted father sued NHS penny pinchers who refused to go on treating her" and found it disgusting, given their assumption that her father had given her one more chance and an extra year of happiness, that "the men in suits who tried to deny her that still claim they were right".[2]

Particularly in the broadsheet newspapers, however, summaries of what had happened in the Child B case were apparently more likely to mention the part that expert medical advice had played in influencing the health authority's decision than they did at an earlier period. Box 16 illustrates how the decision was explained in the main news articles of the newspapers concerned.

Several of the newspapers acknowledged that the positions of both Child B's father and the health authority were understandable and that there would inevitably sometimes be tensions between individual patients (or their advocates) and the bodies responsible for purchasing health care for a population. At the time of Jaymee's death, quite a few journalists argued that the health authority should not be castigated because its decision was appropriate. Several also praised the way its chief executive, Stephen Thornton, had handled the case. The *Daily Telegraph* headlined one article "Grief of caring executive portrayed as the man who said no".[5] The consistency with which the health authority had explained and stood by their original decision was positively portrayed in most broadsheet articles but was presented negatively as unreasonable obstinacy in the *Daily Mirror* and *Sun*.

Channel 4 News devoted the most attention to the issue of Jaymee Bowen's own preferences regarding further treatment. In an interview, Robert Maxwell, chief executive of the King's Fund said that:

> "'In the end, the most important decision is the patient's decision, if it is fully informed' and argued that 'All the signs were that Jaymee was fully informed. No doubt she was influenced by her father, but she knew a lot of what she was taking on, and that's what she wanted. In the end, that's extremely important, albeit the doctors' views are important too'".

Box 16 Broadsheet explanations of the health authority's decision

"Doctors at Addenbrookes said it would not be in her best interests to put her through the ordeal or more chemotherapy and a second bone marrow transplant". (*Daily Telegraph*)[3]

"NHS doctors advised the authority that she should not have a second [bone marrow transplant]. The decision was made in fairness to the child and because the chances of success were deemed to be extremely poor. She was offered palliative medicine to help her symptoms and to allow her to enjoy what remained of her life". (*Daily Telegraph*)[4]

"On the face of it, the death of Jaymee Bowen supports the contention of NHS doctors that extra treatment would have been pointless. In January 1995 . . . they decided that a second operation would serve no useful purpose and would merely put her through unjustified pain and intense radiation doses and chemotherapy. . . . Jaymee's doctors concluded that the probabilities of her benefiting from a second bone marrow transplant didn't stack up. 'We never at any time said we would not pay for her care, but it was not the right thing to do', said Mr Thornton. Logically the NHS line was coherent. Given the constraints of funding it was deemed better value for money to invest £75,000 on the wellbeing of many rather than a high risk pain inflicting attempt to save a dying girl . . .". (*Guardian*)[5]

"Her doctors said that there was no hope and that further treatment might only prolong suffering. . . . The health authority . . . refused because of the pain involved, no one in her condition had ever survived it, and the best experts at the Royal Marsden gave the same second opinion. (The health authority always said they would have paid for any treatment the Marsden recommended.) So it was not entirely a matter of the £75,000 cost. But nor was money absent from their thinking". (*Independent*)[6]

"Mr Bowen refused to accept Cambridge Health Authority's decision that Jaymee's chances of survival were so slim that they did not warrant spending £75,000 on chemotherapy and a possible second bone marrow transplant". (*Times*)[7]

"The treatment was opposed by the 22 NHS centres specialising in childhood cancer on the ground that it was unethical to experiment on a child who was too young to give informed consent. It was for this reason that [the health authority] refused to fund the treatment". (*Times*)[8]

This statement was given some emphasis because it was almost the last word in the main news item (which concluded by arguing that few cases have inspired such fierce debate about rationing, but Jaymee's case was above all a personal tragedy, and noting that she had died without discomfort).

The benefits of treatment

Newspaper articles carried various messages about the benefits or otherwise of the donor lymphocyte infusion treatment. Dr Gravett was quoted in all three television news programmes and several newspapers as being confident that it had given Child B a year of life which she would not otherwise have had. His views were endorsed by Professor Goldman of the Hammersmith Hospital in the *Daily Mail*,[9] and other reports implied this too. Four articles questioned whether the treatment had actually been responsible for Child B living longer than NHS doctors had predicted she would. Box 17 provides a typical selection of statements to the effect that the treatment did prolong her life and the four statements which raised doubts about the causality of the link.

Box 17 Did the experimental treatment prolong Child B's life?

"Yesterday Dr Gravett said Jaymee had been given a year of relatively good health as a result of his care. 'Conventional treatment would have allowed her a few more weeks'". (*Guardian*)[5]

"'She had a very good year and I don't think there is any doubt that she would not have lived so long without the treatment she received'—Professor Goldman". (*Daily Mail*)[9]

"Her sister's healthy blood cells had been used to sustain Jaymee's life for 15 months". (*Sun*)[10]

"Experiment gave pioneer Jaymee an extra year of life". (headline, *Times*)[8]

"No one will know whether the lymphocyte infusion was a factor in her longer survival, for there is no doubt that Jaymee was a great fighter". (*Daily Telegraph*)[4]

continued

"Since she was not part of a controlled trial, no-one will ever know if her treatment gave her the extra year. It might just have been the chemotherapy". (*Independent*)[6]

"Every case has to be taken on its own merits and we will never know if Jaymee would have survived this year without the treatment". (Stephen Thornton, quoted in the *Sun*)[11]

"Experimental treatment like this is a very difficult issue. After all, we do not know whether she would have lived for a year, as she did, without this sort of treatment". (Dr Zimmern, quoted in the *Times*)[12]

Only one of the television news programmes and relatively few newspapers raised the possibility that the donor lymphocyte treatment itself had harmed Jaymee or contributed to her death. Most articles simply reported that she had lost her fight against cancer or leukaemia, and some noted that the leukaemia had relapsed shortly before her death. Channel 4 reported that several doctors had questioned whether the treatment simply prolonged her suffering. The *Daily Mirror* gave a small clue to the fact that the treatment caused problems in a summary history of Jaymee's "6 year battle to beat the big C".[13] The entry for May 16 1996 noted "side effects of treatment make her breathless and tired". The main *Daily Mirror* stories, however, did not attribute any of Jaymee's health problems to the treatment she received.

The *Sun*[10] and *Times*[7] both reported Jaymee's father as saying that the treatment which was keeping the leukaemia at bay had damaged Jaymee's lungs to such an extent that if it had gone on she would have needed a lung transplant, which he was not willing to put her through. Two articles in the *Times*[8,14] also explained the concept of graft versus host reaction in more detail, and one outlined its possible "horrific consequences". It was a feature article in the *Daily Mail*, however, which emphasised the adverse effects of the donor lymphocyte infusion to the greatest extent.[15] Angela Levin, who interviewed Jaymee a few weeks before she died, had quickly discovered that she was terribly ill again, "not this time with leukaemia, but with a horrific side effect of her latest treatment" which had "spiralled out of control and brutally attacked Jaymee's lungs". The journalist was so concerned about Jaymee that she telephoned De Gravett, who explained that it was difficult to be selective with graft versus host disease, which could attack internal organs. He reportedly expressed doubts about his ability to help and said "we are now in danger of substituting one lethal disease for another". The journalist continued:

> "He said they were investigating the cause of Jaymee's painfully swollen face. It might have been caused by a simple infection, but antiobitics weren't working because of the heavy steroids she was taking to help her breathing. It seems steroids were also responsible for her increased body hair. Jaymee was trapped in a vicious medical circle from which, as time soon proved, there was to be only one escape".[14]

Such a specific negative view was notably rare in the media coverage analysed, possibly because few journalists had interviewed Jaymee since she started to suffer from the side effects of the treatment and possibly because they were keen to emphasise the positive aspects of her life, particularly since she was given the controversial treatment. Most articles downplayed the unwanted side effects of the experimental donor lymphocyte treatment, although Jaymee's handling of the "gruelling" treatment was regularly pointed out.

Was it worth it?

The questions of whether Jaymee had ultimately benefited from the treatment Dr Gravett provided and whether the expenditure was justified were raised and discussed in several articles. Some issues were quite thoughtfully considered in individual articles and items.

Assuming that the last 15 months of Jaymee's life could be attributed to the treatment she received, the quality of that extra time had to be considered. Jaymee's father and Dr Gravett were reportedly convinced the time had been good, arguing that she had been able to do "just about anything she wanted", including many things she had never done before. The *Daily Mirror* also used this argument to answer the question "Was it worth it?" in the affirmative, covering a page with pictures of Jaymee swimming, roller skating, returning to school and going on a trip to Calais, and receiving a Children of Courage award from the Duchess of Kent.[16] Similar spreads of pictures in the *Sun*[17] and *Times*[8] also highlighted activities which Jaymee had been able to enjoy. Every newspaper reported at least once that Jaymee's father had told Dr Gravett after Jaymee died, "don't let anyone tell you we failed".

Dr Gravett was widely reported as saying that he would do the same again for another patient in the same situation.

Journalists seemed less willing to talk about the things Jaymee had been unable to do in the months before her death and the difficult times as well as the happy ones. The breathing problems she experienced towards the end of her life, which kept her from school and made crossing the road an ordeal, were mentioned in only three newspapers. Only one article pointed out that she found it hard to swallow and was "thoroughly miserable" about her appearance when she developed thick body hair and a swollen face.[15] Another article was alone in reporting the claim of an expert on acute myeloid leukaemia that it simply was not the case that dying of leukaemia was no worse than dying of the side effects of experimental treatment.[8]

It is obviously difficult to estimate what proportion of the last 15 months of Jaymee Bowen's life was happy, and, not surprisingly, journalists varied in their overall judgments. Statements which Jaymee herself made at different times during the period were quoted in a variety of contexts and frames to give some quite different impressions about the value of the treatment. Box 18 attempts to give some indication of the range of these.

Box 18 Was the treatment worth while?

"'15 months that were the best months of her life' her dad said last night. 'She did lots of things she'd never done before. She went in a stretched limo. She went to France. She read a lesson in Westminster Abbey and they named her Child of the Year'". (*Daily Mirror*)[18]

"Last night, all Britain was asking whether it had all been worth while. Was the authority right in the first place? . . . I think the best answer lies in Jaymee's own words. In a rare interview, she declared 'I would rather go through more suffering to live than to go through no suffering and die'". (*Daily Mirror*)[16]

"Questions have been asked about whether Jaymee had a quality of life which could justify the 437 extra days she lived after the High Court case. It is a difficult question, but there were many, many times when she was genuinely happy. Her favourite day of last year was her eleventh birthday party, when, in the back garden of her Grandparents' home . . . she danced to a steel band and ate ice

continued

cream and cake until she felt sick. She had a few months back at school—schoolwork was crucial to her ever-inquisitive mind—and she even began seeing a boyfriend. Jaymee was not unhappy, although she often insisted in an irritated way that she was not superwoman and that she sometimes got 'totally fed up' of her celebrity status". (*Times*)[19]

"She had her dark moments, when the gruelling treatment that would have worn down a heavyweight boxer held her in excruciating pain. When it all became too much. When she said she really didn't want to carry on. . . . But those moments were rare. The real Jaymee Bowen was the kid who, the day after the court case waltzed around the *Daily Mirror* offices announcing that one day she'd probably be an actress". (*Daily Mirror*)[18]

"'The pain wasn't worth it', Jaymee whispered to me. And, in the end, I'm forced to conclude she was right". (Front page banner headline, *Daily Mail*)[15] "It was only when I was leaving that Jaymee let slip a clue to her innermost feelings. 'I suppose the last time I was really happy was when I was five, before all this started'. In a way, that says it all". (*Daily Mail*)[15]

People's preferences for treatment may vary over time, particularly with their state of health. Some, but not all, articles distinguished between what Jaymee had said about wanting treatment while she was in remission and feeling quite well from what she said nearer the time of her death when she was so debilitated. Five newspapers revealed that Jaymee had said she did not want to go through the treatment again or that she had "already had leukaemia too many times". Without detracting from the sentiment that Jaymee would be remembered for her refusal to give up and her courageous statement that she would rather go through suffering to live than go through nothing and die, her subsequent admission that "there just comes a time when you can't go on with it" was occasionally reported.

The question of the cost-effectiveness of the treatment was, with a few exceptions, largely ignored. Dr Gravett was quoted in four newspapers as saying that £6000 a month was worth paying to have an 11 year old girl running around, while another doctor writing in the *Daily Express* thought that the health authority had been vindicated as "£75 000 is a lot of money to pay for an extra year of a child's life", particularly if the child is likely to die anyway and the money could have produced greater benefit if spent elsewhere.[20] The *Independent* devoted a whole article to discussing the difficulties of valuing a child's life in economic terms.[21]

Was anything else gained from treating Child B?

A few newspaper articles hinted at the question of whether anything was learnt from the experience of treating Jaymee which could benefit future patients. One journalist commented that we would be naive not to realise that if a treatment has not worked on one patient, doctors will at least hope to learn something for the next patient in the queue and said it would be a consolation if the treatment Jaymee received might be refined so that another child might benefit, but she was doubtful whether this would be the case.[15] The *Independent*, consistent with its earlier coverage of the case, pointed out that more would have been learnt if the treatment had been given as part of a coordinated programme of controlled trials. It reported that the chairman of the UK Children's Cancer Study Group said that "if health authorities give in to patient pressure and fund untried expensive treatments outside official trials, trials would be wrecked in popular stampedes with no clear outcomes".[6]

Dr Gravett was reported as claiming several benefits from the publicity given to Jaymee and the treatment he gave her. For example, in the *Daily Mirror* he said that her brave battle had been an inspiration to many other leukaemia victims and had raised the profile of donor lymphocyte infusion[22] (the implicit assumption that this latter was a good thing was not challenged). Several of Dr Gravett's comments also mentioned that the treatment had been worth while from Jaymee's father's point of view. He argued that David Bowen thought he had done everything he possibly could have done, which was important because "if he had given up sooner he would have found that difficult to live with".[6 14 23] He had also "packed a lot into the year he had with Jaymee and it's something he will always remember".[10] A few journalists suggested that the father may have (unconsciously perhaps) been handling his own needs, possibly to the detriment of his daughter.

Box 19 illustrates the range of statements made in the newspapers about what Child B's case would be remembered for. Most of these fall into two categories: the memorability of the character of a remarkable child; and the way the case brought health care rationing to public attention. It is interesting to note that the case was very rarely explicitly seen as highlighting issues surrounding the treatment of seriously ill children or the implications of disagreements between doctors and patients or their advocates.

Box 19 Why will the Child B case be remembered?

"Jaymee will be remembered for her cheeky smile and determination as she stole the limelight while mixing with celebrities in her final year". (*Daily Express*)[23]

"Her case threw into debate the whole question of NHS funding. . . . Jaymee's case has focused attention on the dilemmas facing the NHS in the next decade as medical advances outstrip resources". (*Daily Express*)[23]

"Professor Maurice Lessof of the Royal College of Physicians said Jaymee Bowen's case had reopened the public's eyes to the fact that choices had to be made". (*Daily Express*)[23] (*Independent*)[24]

"Jaymee's case sparked a debate about NHS spending". (*Daily Mail*)[9]

"In her 11 short years of life she suffered 3 bouts of leukaemia, provoked furious rows over the state of the National Health Service, was an inspiration for other cancer sufferers, became the most famous child in the land, and in the end, sadly a guinea pig for medical science". (*Daily Mail*)[15]

"Jaymee was an inspiration for the way she fought leukaemia and the bureaucrats of the health service . . . her memory should inspire us to battle on to save the health service". (*Daily Mirror*)[1]

"Her case not only highlighted the issues surrounding the rationing of health care. It was also the story of a girl facing dreadful odds with courage, resilience and insight". (*Daily Telegraph*)[3]

"Her name was Jaymee Bowen but she will probably always be remembered as Child B. And that pseudonym will probably always be seen as a symbol of youthful determination to live". (*Guardian*)[5]

"She prompted deep soul searching within the health service over its approach to patients diagnosed as terminally ill". (*Guardian*)[5]

continued

"Controversy about the issues in her case will live on for as long as dying patients press for expensive untried treatments against the rigid confines of NHS budgets". (*Independent*)[6]

"Jaymee Bowen brightened all our lives. Her courageous fight against leukaemia was a beacon of hope in a sorry world. And a crushing answer to the charge that kids today don't have what it takes" (*Sun*)[2]

Discussion

At the time of Jaymee Bowen's death, the media not surprisingly devoted space to tributes to the character of the child who had, albeit unwittingly, become a celebrity. They also reflected to some extent on the significance of the Child B case, which they continued to claim had highlighted the issue of rationing in the NHS.

Jaymee Bowen's death resolved the question of what would be the outcome of further treatment which NHS doctors had advised against, which her father had fought for, which Dr Gravett had been willing to provide, and which Cambridge Health Authority had refused to fund: it was not a cure or a particularly lengthy period of remission. The media reported varying opinions about whether, on balance, the treatment had benefited Jaymee and whether it had been worth while, and selectively presented information about aspects of Jaymee's last 15 months of life in support of these.

In the earliest reporting of the case, the contested treatments were further chemotherpy and a second bone marrow transplant. As we reported in the first part of this chapter the clinical considerations which tended to persuade most medical specialists to advise against these treatments were generally played down in the media and particularly the tabloid press, which saw the case primarily as an example of rationing and sometimes presented it as the story of a dying girl being denied a "necessary" treatment. The second bone marrow transplant was never given, and when Dr Gravett announced he would be giving Child B an experimental treatment called donor lymphocyte infusion this was hardly contested in the media (although it seems some journalists asked challenging questions during a press conference).

In retrospect, after Child B's death the newspapers, particularly the broadsheets and one particular feature in the *Daily Mail*, paid far more attention to the arguments against treatment. The role of clinical considerations and medical advice in the health authority's decision not to fund the treatment her father requested was given more prominence than it had in earlier reports. With the exceptions of the *Daily Mirror* and *Sun* the newspapers were generally careful to emphasise the appropriateness of the health authority's decision and the fact that it was not driven by callous financial motivations. Although the newspapers did not explicitly emphasise that the case had exemplified the difficulties of decisions about the treatment of seriously ill children, they nevertheless covered some of these in their reporting.

As we have argued before, in the absence of empirical studies we can only speculate about the impact of media coverage of the Child B case on public perceptions and behaviours. The fact that the two highest circulation tabloids, the *Sun* and *Daily Mirror*, arguably went out on a limb in adopting Child B's cause, persistently standing by their position that she should be given the treatment her father wanted on the NHS, and framing all aspects of the story to fit in with this, however, is worth remarking on.

In their coverage of the Child B case the media provided a highly interesting story about an appealing character. At the time of her death, some reporting was more reflective than had previously been the case about the clinical issues concerned, and was more sympathetic with the position of the health authority and its chief executive who had made the decision not to fund unevaluated treatment for Child B. The Child B case is one that people are likely to remember, and it is likely to live on in future health policy debates.

Part 2 of this chapter was prepared after consideration of comments on the case and on a draft of part 1 provided by Bruce Charlton, Angela Coulter, Alan Maynard, Julian Tudor Hart, Diana Jakubowski, Alison Wick, Alan Williams, and Lewis Wolpert. We are grateful for the insight they shared. This section, however, does not necessarily reflect their views.

1 Anon. A battle worth fighting for. *Daily Mirror* 1996 May 23:6.
2 Anon. Beacon of hope: Jaymee Bowen brightened all our lives. *Sun* 1996 May 23:6.
3 Marks K. One girl's private fight that became a public battle. *Daily Telegraph* 1996 May 23:4.
4 Hall C. Grief of caring executive portrayed as the man who said no. *Daily Telegraph* 1996 May 23:4.

5 Pilkington E, Mihill C. "Never give up unless you are just on the last little drop of life you have in you". *Guardian* 1996 May 23:1–2.
6 Toynbee P. Jaymee and final choices: the story behind the story. *Independent* 1996 May 23:1.
7 Midgley C. "Jaymee was special. She tried so hard and came so close". *Times* 1996 May 23:1.
8 Laurance J. Experiment gave pioneer Jaymee an extra year of life. *Times* 1995 May 23:9.
9 Evans C, Ungoed Thomas J. Don't let anyone tell you that we have failed. *Daily Mail* 1995 May 23:7.
10 Crawford S, Kandohla T. She tried so hard, she came so close. *Sun* 1996 May 23:4–5.
11 Rayner G. We were right to refuse her. *Sun* 1996 May 23:4.
12 Anon. Saddened staff deny that they abandoned girl. *Times* 1996 May 23:9.
13 Anon. Her 6 year battle to beat the big C. *Sun* 1996 May 23:2.
14 Anon. Father's words console consultant who dared. *Times* 1996 May 23:9.
15 Levin A. "It wasn't worth the pain", Jaymee whispered to me. In the end, I'm forced to conclude she was right. *Daily Mail* 1996 May 23:8–9.
16 Anon. Was it worth it? What do you think? *Daily Mirror* 1996 May 23:4–5.
17 Evison S. I don't mind all the suffering if it means a chance of life. *Sun* 1995 May 23:28–29.
18 Reade B. "You tried so hard, love ... you tried so very hard". *Daily Mirror* 1996 May 23:2–5.
19 Midgley C. She wanted to come back as a butterfly. *Times* 1996 May 23:18.
20 Daniels A. Just what price does a doctor put on any life? *Daily Express* 1996 May 23:8.
21 Cooper G. Putting a price on the life of a child. *Independent* 1995 May 23:5.
22 Turner L, Kane P, Wilson E, *et al.* I would do the same again says her doctor. *Daily Mirror* 1996 May 23:5.
23 Hussey M, McGowan B. My fight for Child B was not in vain. *Daily Express* 1996 May 23:15.
24 Cooper G. Child B's treatment worth the money. *Independent* 1996 May 23:5.

The author gratefully acknowledges Liz Cooper, Anne Davies, and Christine Jackson for their substantial contribution to this chapter.

Further details of research reported here can be found in Coope L, Coote A, Davies A, *et al. Voices off: Tackling the democratic deficit in health*. London: IPPR, 1995.

The author also wishes to thank Chris Heginbotham, David Knowles, Shirley McIver and Stephen Harrison for their comments on the first draft.

6 The democratic deficit

ANNA COOTE

Introduction

The British public is deeply interested in health and illness and especially in the NHS. A prodigious amount of TV viewing related to health bears witness to this, with fictional series such as *Casualty* and *Peak Practice* competing with countless documentaries and current affairs programmes. Newspapers and magazines are crammed with reports of crises in the NHS and advice on how to live a healthier life. And nothing is more likely to knit a community together than the threat of a hospital closure.

The actual connection between the public and policy making on health is negligible. Most decisions are taken within a framework set by government or at local levels and by individual health authorities, GP fundholders, and provider trusts. Choices are made and implemented every day of the year. Insofar as they are accountable for their decisions the authorities, GPs, and trusts must answer to the Secretary of State for Health, who in turn answers to parliament. Every four to five years we the public can vote for a new parliament and, possibly, for a new government. This is the only direct power we have to shape decisions about health. Less directly, we elect local authorities, many of which have health committees. Two further mechanisms (non-executive directors of health authorities and trusts, and community health councils) provide limited opportunity for indirect public participation. Beyond that, there is only the power of voice: by protest or persuasion, by opinion surveys or public meetings, we can say what we think. Whether the decision makers hear or heed us is up to them.

Does it matter? In this chapter I argue that public involvement is essential to the process of public accountability which in turn is essential for the NHS. I then consider actual and potential ways in which the public might be involved in decisions about health in general and health care in particular. I am concerned here with decisions about the shape and purpose of services for health, where the issues at stake are more political than clinical in nature.

What is accountability?

John Stewart has suggested that accountability is not guaranteed merely by democratic election; it is a two way process. He distinguishes between *being held to account* and *giving an account*:

> "Both are necessary for the full expression of accountability. Being held to account is enforced through the election and is necessarily periodic. Accounting is equally important to the continuing relationship of stewardship and should involve not just the giving of an account but listening to what is said . . .".[1]

Accordingly, the accountability of a public authority requires a continuing exchange or dialogue with the electorate in which the public can both obtain and provide information, while the authority is open to scrutiny, listens and responds. This process informs the authority's decision making between elections as well as voters' choices at election time. In this way active, participatory democracy may be seen as complementing and validating representative democracy.

Effective accountability demands that responsibilities are clearly located, that those to whom account is given are clearly identified, and that relationships are clearly understood.[2] But clarity in these matters is rare.

Where do responsibilities lie?

The Conservative government's reforms have devolved responsibility to localities and dispersed it within them. Regional health authorities have been abolished. District health authorities and family health services authorities have been merged into local health authorities, planning and purchasing services from semi-autonomous provider trusts. The focus of health care is being shifted from hospitals to community based settings, with the lead given to family doctors. Purchasing power is divided between GP fundholders and local health authorities.

While more and more decisions are taken at local levels, vestiges of local accountability (local councils' nominees on health authorities and boards) have been swept away in the NHS reforms. The responsibilities of the new local health authorities are clearly defined, but they are not directly or demonstrably accountable to their local populations. One effect of the reforms has been a covert enhancement of power at the centre. The convention of ministerial responsiblity, while theoretically respectable, fails to deliver democratic accountability. Stewart *et al* have predicted:

> "A burden is being put upon the accountability of ministers that is probably beyond their capacity to bear. It is difficult enough to expect ministers to accept responsibility for the acts of civil servants who are directly under their own control, without expecting them to extend their responsibilities as is required by the erosion of accountability at local level. It is likely that the increasing burden of accountability on ministers will not be matched by an acceptance of responsibilities".[3]

Members of parliament can deliver little more than a rudimentary form of retrospective accountability through the select committee system and by referring individual cases to the ombudsman. The government's use of patronage to appoint directors to authorities and trusts has remained largely unchallenged by parliament. Meanwhile, market rules and contracts between purchasers and providers tend to exacerbate the problem by encouraging commercial confidentiality rather than open governance.

The problems associated with managing finite resources have become more visible and more urgent as a result of the government's NHS reforms and its efforts to curb public spending. Yet the reforms have fragmented responsibilities and blurred lines of accountability. The Secretary of State and the NHS Executive, local health authorities, GP fundholders, and provider trusts all play a part, directly or indirectly, in setting priorities and allocating resources. Decisions taken by doctors according to their professional judgment about the capacity of individual patients to benefit may now be influenced by purchasers who are concerned with how to get the best "value for money". GP fundholders are expected to apply both sets of criteria—a feat for which their training and professional culture leave them unprepared.

At the macro level, questions of priorities in health care cannot be treated as purely managerial or clinical matters: they affect the population as a whole and the distribution of public funds. They are essentially political questions which need to be settled with democratic legitimacy. Furthermore, if the aim, as government and opposition parties claim, is better health for all rather than just better health services, then decisions about health, including resource allocation, must be integrated with decisions about other public services, such as education, housing, social care, urban and rural planning, environmental services, transport, leisure, and recreation. All have an impact on the health of the nation. Coordinating strategies across traditional departmental boundaries requires strong political direction, exercised by government (national and local) and endorsed by the electorate.

To whom are the responsible authorities accountable?

As a publicly funded organisation providing services for the public in the public interest the NHS is widely acknowledged to owe accountability to the public. But it is important to recognise that the public have a dual role in relation to the NHS. Members of the public are patients and they are citizens. As patients they have an immediate interest in what happens to them as they use or try to use services. As citizens they have a wider interest in how their taxes are spent and in what happens to themselves, their families, and to the wider community, both now and in the future. These two sets of interests may conflict, not least when decisions have to be made about how money is spent.[4] For example, the option of an expensive but potentially lifesaving treatment for one individual may have to be weighed against other options which would benefit a greater number.

Patients have little effective power to call the NHS to account. Despite the development of a quasi market and the arrival of commercial terminology which describes them as "consumers" or "customers", patients have little or no right to choose or "exit" as shoppers in a marketplace. It may be agreed that patients should have more power—for example, extended choices, better access to information, and clear rights to fair treatment. But so long as the NHS remains a public authority, responsible for the health of the whole population, patient power can be no substitute for accountability to the *public as citizens.* Planning for better health for all and for equitable and appropriate health care, with limited resources, is inevitably more than the sum of countless decisions taken by doctors on behalf of their individual patients.

The rest of this chapter examines current and potential strategies for involving the public in commissioning and providing health services: non-executive directors on health authorities; community health councils; Local Voices initiatives; alternative methods of consultation (citizens' juries and electronic democracy); consultations by trusts and GP fundholders; and open governance. Finally, I briefly consider the Healthy Cities initiative and the case for local authorities becoming the commissioning agencies for health.

Non-executive directors of health authorities

Local health authorities are unelected quangos. The only gesture towards local accountability is the appointment of non-executive directors (NEDs) to these authorities. Each has five NEDs and a non-executive chair. They sit alongside five senior officials from the authority, who act as executive directors. NEDs are appointed for up to four years and may be reappointed. They are not (nor have they ever been) required to *represent* the local community; in the post-reform NHS the representative principle is explicit rejected. NEDs are supposedly chosen for their independence, detachment, and skills. At the same time they are expected to provide "accountability through the NHS Executive to ministers and to the local community".[5]

Health authorities have been found to include a low proportion of women and ethnic minorities and an increasing proportion of individuals from private sector backgrounds rather than from public or voluntary service. There is evidence that a large proportion of NEDs have Conservative party affiliations and that they are more likely than executive directors to sympathise with Tory values.[6] They are considered unlikely to mount any serious challenge to the views of the "chair/chief executive duopoly".[7]

District health authorities and family health services authorities formally merged in 1996; the new local health authorities have a more strategic and politically sensitive role than in the past. They are concerned with assessment of needs, purchasing, and contracting, not with direct management of services. NEDs appointed from local communities are supposed to provide "sensitivity" to local needs. Yet nearly one in four such directors lives outside the area covered by the authority.[8] In any case, sensitivity is not, as implied, a satisfactory alternative to accountability. Appointed directors can be accountable only upwards, to those who appoint them. The case for democratic accountability becomes stronger as health commissioning entails increasingly difficult and value laden decisions about priorities and resource allocation. As the Institute for Public Policy Research argues elsewhere,[9] what is required is a clear national framework, setting out criteria and procedures within which locally sensitive decisions can be made.

It has been suggested by the National Association of Health Authorities and Trusts (NAHAT), in its evidence to the Nolan committee, that efforts be made to encourage people from a wider cross section of the community to put their names forward for appointment (from the 1995 report of the association's oral evidence). The BMA has called for a more stringent appointments procedure to restore confidence in the system.[10] In some parts of the NHS attempts have already been made to open up the channels from which NEDs are recruited and to ensure that they are appointed in a relatively open and proper manner. For example, the South and West region advertises appointments, holds open days and roadshows for interested candidates, and interviews candidates and measures them against known criteria of the skills, abilities, and qualities required. They even involve the local community health councils (CHCs) in some appointments.[11]

An independent public appointments commission operating openly with clearly defined objectives and procedures would be an improvement. The Nolan committee has endorsed this idea.[12] There seems to be strong public support for parliamentary scrutiny of public appointments, although it carries a danger of appointments being influenced by trading between political parties.

Useful though such measures may be, none would make health authorities genuinely accountable to local citizens. Arguably, the NEDs could perform a more useful function if it were part of their formal duties to develop a dialogue between local people and their authorities. As the audit commission has suggested, NEDs should cultivate active links with their local communities through public meetings and other consultative measures and through liaison with voluntary sector groups; they should also put pressure on the chairs of their authorities to discuss the implications for the local community of every major decision.[13] The problem with NEDs at present is that they alone speak for the locality on the health authority.

Community health councils

Established by statute in 1974, CHCs are the main official channel for public concerns about the health service. There is one for each local health authority, with some exceptions. They were established and funded by regional health authorities until the latter's abolition—a responsibility which passed to the regional offices of the NHS Executive. Each council has 18 members. Half are appointed by the local authority, one third by the voluntary sector, and the rest by the health regions.

They have no rights of representation on the boards of health authorities or trusts. They are, however, entitled to seek relevant information from the NHS, to have access to certain NHS premises, to meet their health authority once a year, and to be consulted on "substantial developments or variations in service".[14,15] Any objections they have on these matters are referred to the NHS regional offices.

Since 1991 their responsibilities have been expanded and now include working closely with purchasers in identifying local needs, developing purchasing strategies, and monitoring services; monitoring activity within the Patient's Charter from the patients' viewpoint and helping to develop Charter standards and goals; and advising and supporting trusts in seeking patients' views, and monitoring complaints.

They also have a major role in supporting individual complainants, drafting correspondence, checking response times are met, and acting as a complainant's friend or representative during service committee hearings or informal conciliation sessions. The Wilson committee recommended that this role be further enhanced,[16] and a new NHS complaints procedure was implemented on 1 April 1996.[17] The procedure acknowledges the "major role" CHCs already have in supporting individual complaints and states that the government expects this role to continue.[18]

The main responsibility for consulting CHCs lies with purchasing authorities, but they are not obliged to consult if they consider it in the interest of the health service not to do so. Since 1994, GP fundholders have been urged by government to inform CHCs about major contracts, and provider trusts have been encouraged to consult them formally.[19]

The CHCs have many problems in carrying out their roles. They have to cope with the continuously changing face of purchasing authorities and, in some cases, the loss of coterminous boundaries with them. They have to respond to the impact of raised consumer expectations and the consequent increase in patients' complaints. They have to deal with the dilemma that if they join in discussions with purchasers about rationing services they may legitimise unpopular decisions and lose public credibility for their role as patients' advocates. But if they refuse to do so they cannot complain at the outcome.[20] They have to jump to respond to complex consultative documents from the health authorities, with short deadlines. They have to train themselves to do so. They have to resolve the problem of confidentiality, apparently essential to the "internal market", as they move from health authority meetings to provider inspections. They have to face the dilemma of exactly who they represent: Is it primarily service users or the public at large? They have to negotiate uneasy relationships with GPs whose work they wish to monitor while acting as patients' advocates on complaints. They have to choose the right style. If they are confrontational and critical, access may be denied and comments ignored. If they get too close, they may become a tool of the NHS, unable to maintain their objectivity or set their own agenda.[21] They must be "constantly conscious of their dependence on the grace and favour of those they may have a statutory obligation to criticise".[22]

They are expected to carry out all these varied and complex tasks with no more than two or three staff in most districts. They have tiny spending budgets. Council members vary enormously in their capacity, in both ability and time, to contribute to the work of the community health council and receive no remuneration for doing so. Although "community health councils were created by parliament as part of the accountability mechanism of the NHS" (letter from Stephen Dorrell, parliamentary under secretary of state, to all chairs of regional and district health authorities, 14 February 1992), they were given lamentably limited powers and resources to do so.

There are extreme variations in the way they work and how effective they are. Some are overwhelmed with demands from the health authority; most complain that they are marginalised. Some concentrate on helping individual complainants; others work closely with purchasers. CHCs are often dominated by white, middle class, middle aged people, out of touch with and unknown to the wider community. Yet despite the difficulties they face, some are able to fulfil part or all of their responsibilities with a degree of success. Much depends on the history of local relationships and the personality and skills of people concerned.

To be genuinely and consistently effective CHCs require a radical overhaul. They need better resources. Their functions and status must be clarified and their independence assured. They should be more clearly representative of their local communities and their existence better known to the public and within the NHS. Their income, premises, and selection of membership should be independent of the NHS. They need clear rights in relation to authorities, trusts, and GPs: rights to information, to be consulted, to inspect; rights to counsel and represent individuals. CHCs should be able to demand that senior NHS executives report to their meetings. All these things would help build their credibility and authority, which are essential assets. But if such assets are to be sustained the CHCs should themselves be subject to independent monitoring and evaluation. In April 1995 a working party of the NHS Executive published a consultative document on the implications of possible changes to the CHCs. This acknowledged many of the problems and considered mechanisms for monitoring their work but, importantly, proposed no increase in their budgets or their statutory powers.[23] Suitably resourced as well as reformed, CHCs could perform a useful role as lay experts representing local interests in the commissioning of health services. This would not, however, pre-empt the need for a wider dialogue between health authorities and the public.

Local Voices

The Local Voices initiative, launched by the government in 1992, urged health authorities to "give people an effective voice in the shaping of health services locally"[24]; this called for a "radically different approach from that employed in the past" and in particular "a move away from one-off consultation towards ongoing involvement of local people in purchasing activities". Significantly, Local Voices specifically deals with the role of local participation in purchasing as distinct from providing. It concentrates on the need to develop a communication strategy between the "voices of local people and the voice of the health authority".

Several techniques for obtaining local people's views are suggested in the document: public meetings, contributions from local voluntary groups, focus groups, health forums, rapid appraisal, telephone hotlines, surveys of public opinion, patient satisfaction surveys, and complaints procedures. While not meant to be exhaustive, the suggestions cover most of the commonly used techniques of market research. The health authority is exhorted to articulate its views through the media, by the provision of leaflets and newsletters, through well publicised contact points for information, through readable and accessible planning documents and outreach programmes, and by working with GPs as staging posts for messages to and from the health authority.

The intended purpose, as far as it is apparent, is to enhance the credibility of authorities and legitimate their decisions and to help make services more appropriate to local needs. The initiative, however, has been described as "long on exhortation but short on compulsion"[25]; it does not confer any right on local people to participate in major decisions about health.

Authorities are not required to record the activities of Local Voices or their outcomes. There is little pooling or exchange of information by authorities and no central database. They have few opportunities to learn from each other's successes or failures, although there is evidently much to learn. The process has been described as "the unaccountable in pursuit of the uninformed".[26] The recommendations from the NHS Executive "lack any guidance on the means to resolve the inescapable conflict between . . . different viewpoints. Who is right and who is wrong?"[27]

Early evaluation by government identifies good practice but does not specify criteria by which judgments are made. Authorities rated "good" had consulted widely on purchasing plans, made tangible changes as a result, and established arrangements for feedback. Research conducted by the Institute for Public Policy Research found that authorities have used a wide variety of methods, including postal surveys, opinion polls, consultations with specific groups, focus groups, standing panels, and public meetings.[28] They have designated "local voices", variously, as random and stratified samples and as minority groups, interest groups, the voluntary sector, users of specific services, CHCs, GPs, and complete populations. To add to the confusion different authorities use different terms to describe the methods they use.

Costs varied widely and inevitably influenced the breadth and depth of the exercise. Direct costs ranged from £900 for printing an information leaflet (the only specific funding by one authority) to £100 000 over two years for sustained focus group discussions. Full costs were hard to assess because many items were "below the line": these were variously estimated at between two and four times the direct costs.

Some authorities have treated the exercise purely as window dressing, some as necessary but of marginal importance, and others (a minority) as essential to the planning process. Some employed outside experts; others used their own staff. There was no consistency between authorities regarding the purpose of the exercise. Nor was there any shared understanding of the public's dual role as patient/customer and as citizen.

Postal surveys and public meetings have helped to disseminate information about an authority's plans but were found to yield poor levels of response from a self selected "public". Opinion polls produced clearer results from wider samples but offered respondents limited and predetermined options, little or no new information on which to base their views, and no room for dialogue. Face to face interviews with individual people could provide some information and discussion time but only on a one to one basis and within narrow limits. Focus groups provided some opportunity for group discussion on the basis of new information but for limited periods and on terms dictated by the authority. Standing panels offered some continuity of contact and varied according to the methods of contact used. A combination of methods was used by some authorities to help overcome limitations. None enabled members of the public to define the aims of the exercise, the issues at stake, or the methods used.

Some methods clearly suited some objectives better than others. For example, opinion polls could be used to elicit straightforward information from the public which might help to assess local needs; consultations with user groups were helpful in planning specific services, of which the groups had direct experience; focus groups and standing panels offered more in depth and informed discussion, which could help citizens to participate more effectively in planning decisions.

In practice, Local Voices initiatives have been used to consult the public rather than to enable them to participate actively in decisions. Consultations with user groups about specific services, involving the public as patients, were found to be more fruitful than attempts to involve the public as citizens. This was because they could be more clearly focused and were relatively easy to organise; their purpose was more readily understood and accepted by the authorities. Most consultations were confined to fringe issues. Where local people's views conflicted with those of the health professionals they tended to be dismissed as ill informed or mistaken.

A government injunction to health authorities to involve the public in decisions will not necessarily make for more responsive authorities, more democratic planning, or better decisions. But the likelihood would increase if certain ground rules were followed. The purpose of each Local Voices initiative should be clear to all: what issues are at stake, why, and in what capacity the public is being involved. Techniques should be clearly defined, appropriate to the purpose, and consistently used. Adequate resources must be available. Details, including outcomes, should be published and disseminated to the public and within the NHS. Methods and results must be properly assessed and findings pooled so that authorities can learn systematically from each other's experience, and best practice should be identified and spread. Long term, independent evaluation should be part of a programme of continuous development.

Ultimately, though, the greatest threat to effective public involvement may come from efforts to reduce "management" costs in the NHS. By 1996 many health authorities were cutting back their public affairs and community liaison work to meet new injunctions from government to spend "less on grey suits and more on white coats". Effective participation costs money which cannot then be spent directly on health care. Will the public support sustained expenditure on public involvement? That question has not yet been asked, let alone answered.

Alternative techniques for involving the public

Alternative methods for involving the public in health commissioning, as yet untried in Britain, include citizens' juries and electronic democracy.

Citizens' juries involve small groups of citizens, selected to represent the general public rather than any interest groups, who take part in a fully informed and extended discussion to reach a decision on a specific question or set of questions. They take evidence from witnesses, whom they can cross examine, and form smaller working groups to deal with particular problems. They deliberate on the questions with the help of a moderator and are expected to draw conclusions but not to reach a unanimous verdict. The authority which commissions the jury is expected to publicise the findings and either follow the jury's guidance or explain publicly why it has chosen not to do so.

The idea is the subject of a separate study by the Institute for Public Policy Research[29] and has attracted considerable interest from health authorities. The first pilot citizens' jury in the United Kingdom was held in conjunction with the Cambridge and Huntingdon Health Authority in March 1996. Sixteen jurors met over four days within the space of one week and covered three broad questions. (What services should the NHS provide? Who should decide? What criteria should guide decisions?). This jury was part of a wider research project at the IPPR, which explored ways of developing an approach to management of resources in health care based on rights and centred on citizens. Further juries were in the planning stages at the time of writing, including two in Kensington, Chelsea, and Westminster Health Authority that were due to consider the management of risk associated with mental health patients being cared for in the community. An evaluation commissioned by the King's Fund and a report by the Institute on the pilot phase are due for publication in 1996–7.

Electronic democracy implies the use of new communications technologies to involve members of the public in political decision making. Techniques range from relatively low tech radio 'phone-ins to interactive electronic town meetings, involving cable televisions and computer networks. These offer opportunities for extending and enriching democracy but also carry dangers of manipulation, distortion, and reductionism. With electronic models, as with citizens' juries, careful experimentation is essential if authorities are to make the most of the opportunities and minimise the dangers.

GP fundholders and the public

The power of health authorities to purchase health care has been considerably changed by the introduction of GP fundholding. By April 1996 about half of the population in the United Kingdom was registered with GP fundholders, who were purchasing as well as providing health care. In 70-odd "total fundholding" pilots, GPs were purchasing all necessary care. Health authorities provide a framework and are supposed to monitor and regulate fundholders' activities. Some work closely with them; others less so. If accountability is to mean anything, public involvement must relate to the place where power is exercised. It follows that the public ought to be involved in the decisions of GP fundholders as well as in those of health authorities.

Fundholders are statutorily accountable to the NHS Executive through the regional offices, with day to day management contact through local health authorities. Within this framework they are free to spend their funds as they see fit to "achieve the most appropriate care for their patients".[30] According to its published accountability framework, the NHS Executive has three expectations of fundholders. Firstly, they are "expected to publish key documents which relate to the management of their fund", providing copies to the health authority and the community health council and making it available at the practice for consultation with patients. Secondly, they have a responsibility to involve patients in service planning and "are [sic] developing a range of models for involving patients in planning". Thirdly, they "should ensure that they have the appropriate arrangements in place for dealing with patient complaints".[30]

To make sense of what GP fundholders are doing—and not doing—about public involvement it is useful to distinguish between their roles as purchasers and providers. As providers they have a relatively straightforward duty to involve individual patients in full discussions about their condition and treatments, to audit their clinical practice, and to deal with complaints. This is recognised in the third obligation set out in the accountability framework and is not central to the concerns of this chapter. As purchasers, on the other hand, GP fundholders have a broader responsibility to identify and meet local needs, which may require more than doctor–patient dialogue. This is recognised, up to a point, in the first two expectations set out in the accountability framework.

There is no solid evidence of how GPs are "developing models for involving patients in planning". The Royal College of General Practitioners reported in 1993 that only 3% of practices (including non-fundholders) had patient participation groups.[31] Several factors mitigate against successful public involvement with GP purchasing.

One is the ethos of medical training and professionalism. This does not lend itself to democratic dialogue, being based on the medical model of health care which focuses on diagnosis, treatment, and cure of disease or infirmity by qualified experts. Another problem is that ordinary people are often in awe of their doctors, perceiving the doctor–patient relationship as one of adult to child. A study published by the Royal College of General Practitioners found that GPs' patient participation projects were short lived: "in areas of social deprivation people feel somewhat daunted by the doctors and lack confidence to sustain such groups".[32] Some may fear that if they appear troublesome they will be struck off their GP's list. In 1994–5, GPs removed 78 000 patients from their lists.[33]

A third problem is that GPs are wrongly assumed to be a suitable proxy for their patients, while patients are wrongly assumed to be a proxy for the "public": this overlooks the potential conflict between the interests of citizens and service users referred to above. The fundholding initiative was heralded as means of "empowering" patients and communities. This was based on an assumption that GPs could speak on behalf of their patients, protect their interests, and represent their views to the decision makers. Fundholding has made GPs more powerful, but neither their patients nor the public at large have shared in their new power. Family doctors often know a great deal about their patients but only from one limited perspective. What they say cannot be taken as a full or accurate account of the needs of their own patients, let alone the needs of the communities in which they practice.

There is much to be said for GPs developing a more adult to adult relationship with their patients. It is undoubtedly important to involve GPs in planning health care for the areas where they practice—whether or not they are fundholders. But it must be understood that they can speak *about* their patients not *for* them. It would help if CHCs (suitably reformed) had a more constructive involvement in fundholders' decision making. Fundholders interviewed for this research observed that their relationship with CHCs was purely adversarial; the councils were the people who took them to court and had no statutory right to "come into primary care". It is doubtful, however, whether GPs themselves will ever be a satisfactory channel for citizen involvement in planning and purchasing decisions—just as it is doubtful whether they are ideally suited to be purchasers. The tasks of identifying population needs and managing finite budgets across a range of competing demands are essential to the purchasing role in today's NHS. There is a fundamental contradiction between this and the essential clinical function of doing everything possible for the individual patient on a case by case basis.

Provider trusts and the public

While hospital and community trusts are constituted as separate provider organisations within the NHS, they should reasonably be expected to maintain a continuing and constructive dialogue with their patients about the way services are delivered. If they also establish a dialogue with the *public as citizens* in their surrounding communities this may be considered as good practice but not, arguably, as an essential duty. It is up to the purchasers to identify needs and secure services to meet those needs.

These distinctions, however, are not clear cut. For one thing, the public evidently perceives the NHS in terms of hospitals and clinicians rather than managers and purchasing authorities. The focus of public attention is on the providers. The policies of provider trusts may also be highly influential in shaping the policies of purchasers: the tail may wag the dog. The trust can take decisions to develop specialisms or to change procedures (for example, to introduce more day surgery) which offer health authorities and GP fundholders new opportunities for allocating their resources.

How, if at all, do the trusts relate to the public? They have NEDs on their boards in the same way as health authorities. Some trusts have close and constructive relations with their local CHCs, but, according to one senior NHS spokesman, many of them "despise community health councils as ineffective and weak" and have little or no understanding of the patient/citizen dichotomy (personal communication). Many trusts have developed their own ways of consulting the public, with varying effects. They commonly use simple patient satisfaction surveys and public meetings, although some have developed more sophisticated methods. Bradford Community Trust, for example, is a member of a local "Speak Out Panel", set up in conjunction with the local authority, health authority, and Training and Enterprise Council, to sample the views of the local population on a regular basis. Community trusts, which provide mental health services, community nursing, and other community based services, tend to have a culture more conducive to user involvement than do acute hospitals trusts. In the latter, where the ethos and interests of senior clinicians predominate, the medical model of health care and doctrine of clinical autonomy sit uneasily with most forms of patient or citizen participation. A report for the former Wessex health region noted that "some clinicians expressed strong reservations [about consumer involvement], anticipating possible breaches of confidentiality".[34]

As a rule it is clinical confidentiality that doctors wish to protect. Managers, on the other hand, are more likely to be concerned with commercial confidentiality. The idea of "listening to local voices" sits uneasily with the trust structure in the NHS. Trusts can in principle (if not often in practice) provide services for any area and operate in a competitive market where commercial confidentiality is increasingly valued. This militates against public involvement and open decision making.

Open governance

Accountability depends on openness. With a complex subject such as health not only must information be made available it must be made comprehensible. Health authorities are obliged by law to publish their annual reports, audited accounts, a five year strategy document, contracts with providers, and the papers and minutes of board meetings held in public. Many of these are opaque and indigestible documents, full of acronyms and language unfamiliar to the general public,[35] although some health authorities produce summary documents which are more accessible and more widely distributed.

Health authorities are subject to the Public Bodies (Admission to Meetings) Act 1960, which requires that their main board meetings are open to the public, but the public may be excluded from "private sessions". The code of practice on openness in the NHS ostensibly aims to ensure that people "are provided with explanations about proposed service changes and have an opportunity to influence decisions on such changes". Yet it lists information which the NHS does not have to provide, including:

> "Information about internal discussion and advice, where disclosure would harm frank internal debate, except where this disclosure would be outweighed by the public interest. Management information, where

disclosure would harm the proper and effective operation of the NHS organisation. . . . Information which could prejudice negotiations or the effective conduct of personnel management or commercial or contractual activities".[36]

The introduction of market rules with provider trusts competing for business and the removal of local government appointees from health authorities have combined to reduce public access to health service meetings and papers. At a recent conference a civil servant told his audience of senior NHS managers not to worry too much about the code. They would "not have to manage in a gold fish bowl", he said, but just be prepared to release information in aggregate form.[37] The NHS code is weaker than the code which applies to central government bodies. It does not apply retrospectively. It does not allow the ombudsman to recommend that exempt information be disclosed in the public interest. It allows all information about commercial or contractual activities to be withheld thus removing the basis of the NHS internal market reforms from scrutiny.

The NHS Executive has begun to publish league tables based on the performance of health authorities measured against indicators from the Patient's Charter. These show, for example, how waiting lists compare from one area to another. Such "openness" is of limited value to the public if individuals remain powerless to influence the quality of care available to them.

The staff of the NHS are constrained in their ability to speak openly about NHS matters. The *Guidance for staff on relations with the public and the media* was distributed in June 1993 with an accompanying executive letter from Sir Duncan Nichol which professed to "encourage a climate of openness and dialogue within the NHS" but expressed a clear preference for staff having "their concerns effectively resolved without the need to go outside the NHS".[38] An internal system to resolve complaints and conflicts is obviously desirable. The guidance seems, however, to confuse the obvious need for the confidentiality of individual patient records with confidentiality in general. It states that "Employees . . . have an implied duty of confidentiality and loyalty to their employer", which is not absolute if the disclosure is made in the public interest. Such justification, however, "should be soundly based" and "if entered into unjustifiably, could result in disciplinary action and might unreasonably undermine public confidence in the Service". In a handful of cases, NHS whistleblowers have been suspended or sacked and the restriction on their freedom of speech justified in the name of competition. Sir Gordon Borrie QC, who is chair of the organisation Public Concern at Work, has observed that employees are given the impression that their job prospects may be jeopardised if they allege malpractice and that this creates "a culture of secrecy, intimidation and coercion where those who speak up are victimised".[39]

Public bodies disbursing public funds should be open to public scrutiny. Commercial practices and patient confidentiality both encourage secrecy, and there is little attempt to safeguard openness in the public interest. The media are often regarded as adversaries to be kept at bay, rather than as allies to assist in disseminating information. The public must be able to judge the performance of their representatives, to understand the issues at stake, and to form their views on the basis of full information. A change of rules and a change of culture are required.

Healthy Cities

A different culture prevails in the European Healthy Cities project. This was set up by the World Health Organisation (WHO) as part of a wider initiative launched in 1977 to achieve "health for all" by the year 2000. Glasgow signed up in 1988 and became one of four pilot cities in the United Kingdom, along with Liverpool, the London Borough of Camden, and (until 1992) Belfast. The WHO defines health as "a state of complete social, mental and physical well-being and not merely the absence of infirmity".[40] Accordingly, health is determined by a range of factors, including employment, housing, transport, access to goods and services, opportunities for leisure and recreation, and the quality of social relationships. This is a "social" model of health, as distinct from the "medical" model described above, and it assumes that responsibility for health must be shared between agencies, not left to the NHS.

Public involvement is central to the Healthy Cities model of health promotion. A leading public health consultant has observed that the model focuses on "the role of government in creating policies and environments supportive of health and in enabling people to increase control over their health through involvement in the process of governance"; it is "fundamentally about democracy in the city" (T Hancock, symposium on Health and the Urban Environment, Manchester, 1994).

In Glasgow, as part of the Healthy Cities agenda, community conferences are held every 12–15 months with a steering group representing more than 20 statutory and non-statutory agencies; recent conference themes have been Gender and Health and Social Justice and Health. In Drumchapel, one of the city's most deprived areas, community health volunteers are recruited and trained to work with self help groups, to run a community health library, to deal with the media, and to join local forums concerned with drugs, nutrition, and other issues. A community support unit, set up in 1992, employs lay health workers who are trained at Strathclyde University and then liaise with local communities to develop their own health strategies.

In a linked WHO led scheme, Sheffield Health for All was set up in 1987. This has involved intensive user group consultation to produce a discussion document, *Our City—Our Health* (1991), leading to a multi-agency agenda to improve people's health. Funds dispensed as part of the scheme have helped the development of a range of projects including work with women, ethnic groups, older people, and children and on issues ranging from mental health, nutrition, and traffic pollution to smoking and assessment of needs—the latter involving large scale questionnaires, structured interviews, focus groups, and other techniques.

Hancock has pointed out that while "we have a system of government that is essentially based on the 19th century . . . a new management style is emerging consistent with the Healthy Cities approach: influence versus authority, power with rather than power over; negotiation not directives, holistic rather than sectoral, both/and instead of either/or" (T Hancock, symposium on Health and the Urban Environment). This sounds encouraging, but in practical terms Healthy Cities and the UK Health for All Network have had no impact on the health status of local populations, although it may be too early to expect anything measurable. More importantly, they have had no serious impact on health policy making, either nationally or locally; even in the cities directly involved the effect has been slight. Statutory agencies are not geared to the WHO model of health development nor are conventional government approaches to health policy. That health has a multiplicity of determinants (including socioeconomic factors), that citizen empowerment is a route to health gain, and that interagency cooperation is essential—these ideas may be widely accepted intellectually but they seem to have little resonance among those with power to change or protect the status quo. A senior Glasgow official has commented that without direct access to the very top of the current statutory agency structures all the will in the world cannot make things happen (Lyon A, personal communication).

The Healthy Cities project is closely allied to the community development model of social welfare, prevalent in the 1970s, debunked in the 1980s, and almost forgotten in the 1990s. It has produced several innovative projects which may yet bear fruit in terms of health gain. It suffers from an organisational and political environment that is apathetic at best and often downright hostile. More radical changes will be required before it can be translated into tangible benefits.

A role for local government?

One such radical change which deserves consideration is to place health commissioning within the ambit of local representative democracy by extending the role of local authorities.

Health authorities undoubtedly depend on local government for the successful implementation of policy, particularly regarding community care and health promotion. This dependence is likely to increase. Joint working between health and local authorities is well established, but the boundaries between, for example, public health and environmental health, and social care and health care, make little sense and can work against effective delivery of appropriate services. The commissioning of health services according to locally determined priorities, together with other public services which have an impact on health, is an appropriate subject for a multifunctional, publicly accountable, representative body.[41,42]

The poor reputation of a few local councils is often used to justify further centralisation of public services. Yet there is evidence that the public attaches greater value to local government than to central government.[43,44] Many councils are now pursuing reforms which will not only deliver better services to users but will also enable people to participate more fully as citizens.[45] Local democracy is being revitalised by changing the way local councils work.

The use of localities by health authorities runs parallel with the trend towards decentralisation in local government. This is characterised by devolution of management decisions, localisation of services, democratisation by increasing participation through neighbourhood forums, and integration by working across service boundaries. Decentralised local government offices would allow differentiated purchasing by localities within a unified plan approved by locally elected councils, the whole being subject to national targets and standards laid down by the Secretary of State answerable to parliament.

Health and health care commissioning within such a structure would require the following features: a population based rather than practice based perspective; involvement of primary health care professionals; responsiveness to local needs and wishes; and a capacity to influence services provided by trusts. By commissioning services to promote good health and treat ill health through decentralised local government, public accountability would be increased in a number of ways. Councillors would be involved at both neighbourhood and council levels. Audit arrangements and access to the ombudsmen (health service and local government) would continue, and accountability to parliament would be obtained through the responsible Secretary of State. A national framework setting out criteria and procedures to guide local decisions (mentioned earlier) would help to offset any danger of increased local democracy undermining the national character of the NHS.

This is an idea which needs to be tested carefully before any conclusions are reached about its viability. A wholesale transfer of health commissioning to local authorities would be impracticable and potentially catastrophic. Enabling legislation could be introduced to allow for a pilot scheme. This would provide a "whole population" or "total district" alternative to the total GP fundholding scheme currently on trial. It would involve GPs in the commissioning process, possibly with indicative rather than with discreet budgets. A handful of authorities could be selected for the pilot where there is a proven record of working closely with the health authority and where suitable plans are submitted.

In respect of spending powers, participating authorities would operate within the same restraints as the present health authorities. Powers to supplement national allocations with local spending or transfer of funds between health and other services (for purposes of preventive health for example) would be considered at a later stage. Without fundamental changes to present rate restrictions, local councils would have no powers to raise local taxes which could offset shortfalls in national funding.

The participating authorities would be charged with the duty to make an assessment of local health needs; to produce an integrated health and social care plan; to make explicit its priorities and any rationing policy; to commission health services according to contracts or service level agreements with providers; to produce an integrated health promotion strategy, which incorporates council policies on housing, education, transport, leisure, and all other areas; and to consider the impact of all policies on health. Last but not least, they would be expected to enter into a genuine dialogue with local citizens as part of the planning process. If, after full evaluation, the pilot scheme were deemed a success, the model could be extended to more authorities. If not, it should obviously be scrapped. In any event, combined locality based commissioning of health services would not pre-empt the need for continuing public involvement in health policy development between local elections.

In conclusion

In this chapter I have considered accountability in relation to health policy making: what it entails, who is accountable, and to whom. I have reviewed a range of ways in which the public can be involved in policy decisions. There is no ideal formula. All of the models reviewed are probably worth retaining as part of a "democratic repertoire" at the disposal of commissioning authorities—whether these are appointed health quangos or elected local council.

If each authority were clear about the purpose of involving the public in each exercise it undertook and if it were well informed about what could be achieved by different methods, it could then match purpose to method in appropriate ways. There would be fewer opportunities to waste resources on futile procedures. There might be less cynicism about the authorities' intentions and about the worth of public involvement. It might be possible for citizens to make informed and considered judgments on a range of major as well as minor health issues. If so, it would help to strengthen democracy and to improve the quality of decision making across the country.

1 Stewart J. *Innovations in democratic practice.* Birmingham: Institute of Local Government Studies, 1995.
2 Bartram B. *Accountability check list.* London: Consumer Congress (in press).
3 Stewart J, Lewis N, Longley D. *Accountability to the public.* London: European Policy Forum, 1992.
4 British Medical Association. *Rationing in action.* London: BMJ Publishing, 1993.
5 Department of Health. *Code of conduct. Code of accountability: corporate governance in the NHS.* London: Department of Health, 1994.
6 Ashburn L, Cairncross L. Membership of the "new style" health authorities: continuity of change? *Public Administration* 1993;**71**:Autumn.
7 Ferlie E, Ashburner L, Fitzgerald L. Corporate governance and the public sector: some issues and evidence from the NHS. *Public Administration* 1994.
8 Blunkett D. Answer to parliamentary question. *Guardian* 1994 August 16.
9 Lenaghan J. *Rights and rationing in health care.* London: Institute for Public Policy Research (in press).
10 British Medical Association. *Accountability in the NHS: a discussion paper.* London: BMJ Publishing, 1994.
11 Cooper L, Coote A, Davies A. *Voices off: tackling the democratic deficit in health.* London: Institute for Public Policy Research, 1995:38.
12 Nolan Committee. *Standards in public life.* London: HMSO, 1995 (Cm 22850–1.)
13 Audit Commission. *Taken on board. Corporate governance in the NHS: developing the role of non-executive directors.* London: Audit Commission, 1995.
14 *Community Health Councils Regulations 1995 (SI 1985 No 304) as amended by Community Health Council (Amendment) Regulations 1990 (SI 1990 No 1375).* London: HMSO, 1990.
15 *Community Health Councils (Access to Information) Act 1988.* London: HMSO, 1988.
16 Review Committee on NHS Complaints Procedures. *Being heard.* London: Department of Health, 1994.
17 NHS Executive. *Report.* London. NHS Executive, 1995. (EL(95)37.)
18 Department of Health. *Acting on complaints.* London: Department of Health, 1995.
19 NHS Management Executive. *Report.* London: NHS Management Executive, 1994. (EL(94)4.)
20 Joule N. *Partners in purchasing? The role of the Community health council in commissioning health services.* London: Greater London Association of Community Health Councils, 1993.
21 Buckland S. Community health councils: an effective mechanism for representing consumers in the NHS? *Research, Policy and Planning* 1993;**11**.
22 Jobling R. Reins tighten for future CHCs. *Health Service Journal* 1990;Feb.
23 NHS Executive. *Report of the working group on the implications of the change in establishment arrangements for community health councils.* London: NHS Executive, 1995.
24 NHS Management Executive. *Local voices, the views of local people in purchasing for health.* London: NHS Management Executive, 1992.
25 Rathwell T. A voice in the wilderness. *Health Services Journal* 1992;Oct 29.

26 Pfeffner N, Pollock A. Public opinion and the NHS: the unaccountable in pursuit of the uniformed. *BMJ* 1993;**307**:
27 Salter B. Politics of purchasing in the NHS. *Policy and Politics* 1993;**21**.
28 Heginbotham C. *Listening to local voices.* London: National Association of Health Authorities and Trusts, 1993.
29 Stewart J, Kendall E, Coote A. *Citizens' juries.* London, Institute for Public Policy Research, 1994.
30 NHS Executive. *Accountability framework for GP fundholding: towards a primary care led NHS.* London: NHS Executive, 1993.
31 Pritchard P. *Partnership with patients.* 3rd ed. London: Royal College of General Practitioners, 1993.
32 Heritage Z, ed. *Community participation in primary care.* London: Royal College of General Practitioners, 1994. (Occasional paper No 64.)
33 Committee of Public Accounts. *General practitioner fundholding in England. 27th Report.* London: HMSO, 1995.
34 Barnard S. *Whose audit?* Portsmouth: Social Science and Research Unit, University of Portsmouth, 1995. (Report No 29.)
35 Adam S, Gill M. Paperchase. Health Services Journal 1994;March.
36 NHS Executive. *Code of practice on openness in the NHS.* London: NHS Executive, 1995.
37 NAHAT. *Report on conference on rationing—getting it out into the open.* London: National Association of Health Associations and Trusts, 1994.
38 NHS Management Executive. *Report.* London: NHS Management Executive, 1993. (EL(93)51.)
39 Borrie G. *Health Services Journal* 1993;Nov/Dec.
40 World Health Organisation. *Healthy cities project.* Geneva: WHO, 1990.
41 Harrison S, *et al. Health before health care.* London: Institute for Public Policy Research, 1994.
42 Harrison S, Hunter D. *Rationing health care.* London: Institute for Public Policy Research, 1994.
43 Rallings C, Temple M, Thrasher M. *Community identity and participation in local democracy.* London: Commission for Local Democracy, 1994.
44 Travers T. Can local heroes convince a nation? *Independent* 1995 February 4.
45 Burns S, Hambleton R, Hoggett P. *The politics of decentralising: revitalising local democracy.* London: Macmillan, 1994.

The Partner:

The Institute of Health Service Management

The Question:

How might information technology transform the shape of health services?

The Writer:

Dr John Spiers, President, the Patients' Association

Think Tank Members:

Professor Tony Cullyer, Professor of Economics and Deputy Vice Chancellor, University of York

Dr Paul Hodgkin, General Practitioner, Sheffield, Advisor to the FACTS (Framework for Appropriate Care throughout Sheffield) project

Mr Roy Lilley, Past Chairman, The Homewood Trust, and Independent Health Care Policy Consultant

Professor Marshall Marinker, Visiting Professor of General Practice, UMDS, London and Advisor in Health Care Policy and Medical Education, MSD Ltd

Ms Carole Mortimer, Director of Medical Computing

Rabbi Julia Neuberger, Chairperson of the Camden Community Health Care Trust

Mr Ray Rowden (Chair), Director of the Institute of Health Service Managers

7 "Only a novel!" Jane Austen, hyperspace and the story of patient power

JOHN SPIERS

Souls, silhouettes, scalpels, and sensibilia

We are an unusual generation. We can already look back at our present, and judge it in terms of the nearby digital future. We can look back from our virtual future and ask who we are and who do we want to be. We can inhabit this future virtually, and call it for inspection—from virtual reality to personal *actualité*. We can project ourselves, both within and without. To do so and to make judgments, we need a philosophy of society, a philosophy of technology, and a philosophy of information. Digital realities may empower searches for public policy solutions.

Interactive multi-media will transform British society and public culture, and thus dramatically change the perceptions and expectations of individuals for more autonomy and choice. They have the potential to change both the psychology and practice, the character of health care institutions, and the tasks and limits of government. New connections have the capacity especially to support self-management, in mutual but voluntary co-operation with others. But not all the questions or the answers are obvious. It is not obvious that the digital revolution will necessarily empower the individual, and renovate health care. We need to discuss how this might be achieved, to examine the institutional arrangements and contexts that give activities meaning, to consider the constraints and possibilities of this new context, and to reconcile changes with the need for re-assurance and community.

We are now each virtually global in reach. We are digital. We expect to be empowered to live our own lives, and to benefit quickly from the technical advances of medicine. Yet two contrary worlds co-exist. In the wider world outside medicine, information is transparent; in the narrower world of the NHS it is opaque. NHS information—instead of serving as the currency of connection, activity and value—remains weak and closed. Services are dispensed to powerless patients. Self-command is discouraged. Empowerment is distant, treatment uncertain, even professionally-determined outcomes surprisingly varied. "Disease" is "scientific", and "objective"; but "illness" remains personal and lonely, even for the autonomous individual. And, as Flaubert remarked of doctors: "They cannot find our souls with their scalpels."

There is a habit of ignoring the obvious. What has been most missing in this universe of enquiry is the patient's voice and sense of personal self. The individual and collective unconscious has not been accessed. The notion that the service would like to know what people want is contradicted by what is provided. There is a hierarchical NHS of controls. What is required, instead, are gateways to what patients say. For what counts most to the individual is their position relative to power, their contact with themselves, their potential to accomplish their goals. Decentralisation within NHS structures—location, diversity, vitality—does not necessarily put these goals within individual reach. The difficulties of social consent and legitimacy of NHS Trusts and purchasing authorities document this, since they remain centrally controlled within themselves. There could be an entire re-orientation of the NHS, to position itself in relation to what it hears and learns. The question is how to achieve this.

People and users (or patients, in the medicalised language) have many stories to tell. This is so even when they do not necessarily know what these are or how to tell them. It is necessary to construct a frame of mind and a frame of action which offers these stories, pathways, avenues for expression. By these patients will enter into discourse what they want to say. The need is for intelligence gathering, to get people to tell what is otherwise unknown and unheard. Here, a useful and suitable language and a vocabulary is missing. Thus, the mandate of the NHS is contingently inadequate. The need is for "letter-boxes", for listening devices, as John Simmonds has said. And there are two responsibilities in civil association once this information is invited and collected: to be clear what to do with the evidence, and to respond to the people who provide it. This is to probe a big general question: how can we know what is going on in society? How do we test it? How do we do something about it? Voting is too generalised, too unspecific, too infrequent, too diffuse, too limited in its "choices". Satisfaction surveys have very limp utility. "Consultation" has hardly caught attention. There is an alternative, however, to the sense of placid incomprehension and resigned Asian distraction which Paul Theroux noticed in *The Great Railway Bazaar*, and which remains characteristic of the "chugging locomotive" which is the NHS. One way to test what goes on is to collect information about what people experience, what they say about what happened to them. This is to use technologies to open doors and windows to encourage people to tell the service (and one another) about their experiences. This requires recognition of distinctive identity, and respect for the riddle of the individual, which strengthens the development of forms of common life, and which pre-supposes the value of choice and its companion, which is responsibility. In this we express our vision of the world, define the realm of discussion, name those commitments to which we are most deeply committed. The question of how to make this count, of which devices will ensure empowerment, also needs clear enquiry.[1]

This is to emphasise "narrative". For narrative (like the novel) is a major point of reference in a society and in an individual life. It is a tribunal and a signpost, a definition and a debate. Communities are shaped by the shared experiences of the people in physical communities, in intellectual communities, in imaginative communities, in common social experiences. It is important to talk about these experiences openly, and to reveal the ideas, the sense, the sensibilities we share. This is to place an emphasis on those facts and moral ideas we need to take seriously and personally. This is a decision about how these important moral ideas ought to be highlighted and set up for reference and appeal. We need to set up these ideas, then place a value on open information, then go after it. This is something very significant worth having. We need a concerted effort to get it. Such an ambition asks us to re-examine critically the ends of the system, of each individual, the nature of the organisation, its life and efforts. The NHS needs to be *about* intelligence and data and evidence. It needs, too, to respect the duality of "inside" and "outside". As Paul Theroux wrote, his travel animated by imagination: "I travelled easily in two directions, along the level rails while Asia flashed changes at the window, and at the interior rim of a private world of memory and language. I cannot imagine a luckier combination."

As Angela Coulter has stressed, patients do want to hear from one another. They want to hear what other patients say. People want to learn from the experience of others, and to pass on their own experiences. Questions differ depending on who is asking them. The task is to change the questions into those consumers ask. To change the focus and the language. And for these changes to lead the research agenda, with an awareness of how people live and feel. An individual asks what is the problem, the disease, the possible solutions? The real question is usually whether the treatment proposed will make me better. Will it take the pain away, help me get back to work, let me sleep, keep me safe and well. Medicine seeks to restrict the possible answers to a range of interventions and alternatives. Too many outcomes are professionally defined. The key is to ask about the aims, about how evidence is gathered, about how it is collated, and how effects are measured—from which points of view. People ask different questions: Am I alone? How does my experience compare with that of others? How did they feel about their care, their tests, and the purpose, results, and value of them? Which information would have made them feel easier, and empowered? Did the therapy relieve the symptoms? What were the side-effects? Did it work? What were the effects on their feelings and emotional life? Was it essential to have treatment? What is the natural history of the disease? What was the whole process like? Did professional outcomes coincide with yours? People do want to discover what other people did and experienced when faced with difficulties and with different treatment choices. People do want to know the controversies, the certainties and uncertainties, the gaps in knowledge. They do want a measure for things—for example the orgasm outcome, or what could leave me with a happy and thriving baby—that professionals do not necessarily measure. Patient-defined outcome measures include anxiety, stress, pain, and whether the problem was solved, and what the whole process did to the individual. This is, as John Gray has said, for people "to make their own choices and to be at least part authors of their own lives, in all of the institutions and practices of contemporary liberal societies."

We are a nation of poets and of ambiguity. Yet one which, paradoxically, has preferred bio-medical explanations which are out of balance with our interior intuitions. This perspective has marginalised our psycho-social "reality", and understated our capacity for self-knowledge, judgment and choice. It has disbelieved in what we know about what has happened to us. It has discouraged the development of a public vocabulary with which to discuss difficult issues. Both patients and medical professionals have experienced what Marshall Marinker (citing T. S. Eliot) refers to as a "dissociation of sensibility".[2] The bio-medical emphasis has supported the myth that there is an objective and effective therapy for every condition for every patient. This medicalised idea—which Tony Hope has called "the protocol presumption"—is now being re-emphasised by medicine, yet its evidence base is not rooted in evidence from patients.[3] The protocol idea is the home of hidden value judgments. It exaggerates the powers of "medical expertise". It is uninviting, too, for our expectations of individual human potential, not least because of the epidemiological emphasis on "populations". There are problems, too, about the doctor–patient conversation. Doctors are trusted for the information they give, yet often have poor communication skills. They are, too, susceptible to the "framing effect". They often underestimate the needs of people for information and for time to consider. Social status, context, time-frame, anxiety are all in the way.

In these explorations I offer a view about nature, character, and the sources of social solidarity. The digital revolution is the stile to the next field. It offers a prospectus for responsive care, for user empowerment, for organisational change, for psychological and organisational change. This will be led by the implications of listening with interactive, multi-media, information technology—which no government directs or controls. Fundamentally, this is both a psychological and a practical change. There is an architectural chasm to cross, to connect the potentials to what actually goes on. It will be necessary for the NHS to much improve the quality and integrity of its data as well as to change its cultural assumptions. There are multiple points of failure even when measured against the old problem-definitions of the NHS: inconsistent software and hardware; inadequate accountability and support; high management costs; a lack of end-to-end solutions both for legacy and for new applications. Some 90 per cent of the deficit is in software, the intelligence in the system. This must be renovated, based in standards set directly in close contact with service users and citizens who are future patients and who should pose the questions they want answered. The walking companion is better care.

We have accepted from René Descartes and Francis Bacon the logical reasoning of empirically deductive science. This has closed out other kinds of reasoning, knowledge and expertise, and concealed the truth of what and whom expertise represents. It should be recovered as we revise what we mean by "knowledge" and "expertise". As T. S. Eliot wrote in *The Rock*: "Where is the life we have lost in living? Where is the wisdom we have lost in knowledge? Where is the knowledge we have lost in information?"

New interactive multi-media technologies are social gunpowder. There is a global mobility of information. Relationships, which are key in medicine, will without doubt change a great deal. Medicine will become a three-way relationship: you, me, the machine data. This will be a mutual learning experience, about cost, access, location, narrative stories, international experience, specialisation, quality of life, likely outcomes in a world of economic and social globalisation for which we are, as yet, ill-prepared in our politics and in our health systems. The sharpest report as the fuse burns will be a fundamental enquiry about moral agency, free choice, individual and personal self-reflection and self-responsibility. This is to ask for a stronger—even a compelling—individual voice about individual service and health service development. It implies an appropriate exit to alternatives (within the system or outside it), and information and devices to achieve both.

The liberal view of human potential and enriched autonomy places its emphasis on the bonds of unity which asks each of us to be a custodian of our culture. On this view, the community changes and grows, in touch with shared values for which each of us is responsible. "Community" is not merely the political process, but a personal duty. Marshall Marinker has emphasised, too, that post-modern reality offers more than one reality. It is for individuals to choose theirs, in shared and supportive tolerance.[4] This is not only a difference in reality at the level of DNA, or at the level of the tax-payer. It is a difference at the most intricate psycho-social level, where each of us decides "Who am I?" Health care decisions are increasingly made by reference to this question. Patients are capable of making many such decisions. There are many situations where the patient is genuinely in a satisfactory position to make a decision. Where outcomes are not clear-cut the doctor can try to estimate the risk but the patient has to and can judge its acceptability.

These are not technical questions—and not appropriate areas for paternalistic decision-making. Here, the patient can be the judge of what the information means for them, and which criteria are relevant. There is a moment here when the vital thing to exclude is "expertise", once good information has been offered on negative and positive possible effects.[5]

This appreciation of the importance of coping strategies poses, too, an important choice about "voice" at the organisational level: what do we want the system *to be*? This is essentially a question about human character and potential which the organisation should support. It is a question which will become very pressing politically and voting behaviour will change what politicians ask of the NHS. Health care systems seem increasingly likely to restrict access, as they struggle to mediate "founding values", medical innovation, demographic pressures, professional or patient autonomy, compelling costs, social consent and politics. The re-distributive role will reduce; the stress on quality will be strong and insistent.[6]

Medicine remains innately and unavoidably uncertain. Where patients can decide for themselves between uncertain paths they should be informed and helped to do so if they wish to decide. Yet it is difficult for the individual patient to see a preferred path. There are deliberate assymetries of power and information, differential knowledge and social power. Information about the quality of service and of care remains impoverished and elusive. Medical professionals have appealed in terms of "mystery" and over the heads of rationality and management with special claims to "expertise" and autonomy. This has contradicted the openness required in a public system, and deliberately constrained choice about alternatives and quality. This has been contrary to fairness and equity. It remains a challenge both to the consumer and the citizen. Self-regulation by medical professionals remains unsatisfactory, too, with practice varied, differences in practice-styles unexplained, harmful treatments persistent; there is a need for tighter supervision if optimal practice is to be ensured.[7] Doctors have presented themselves successfully as being without self-interest. In concert with government they have suppressed both information and choice.[8] Governments have continued to work with veto-organisations, in a political marketplace greatly influenced by organised special interests. Medicine is thus politicised and health medicalised.[9] One consequence is that the individual remains in a weak position, both as consumer and citizen, in terms of democratic control over "strategy" and of personal control over own body, own illness, own self. In addition, existing consultative mechanisms concerned with service planning have remained inimical to "involvement", and local accountability.

Can this change? The complicating opportunity is digital. This is a challenge to the axis of the NHS, which is one of corporatist "planning" and "strategy". It will be the challenge of the individual voice. As Seamus Heaney writes, "The piper coming from far away is you."[10] In the era of the electric (if still invisible) hospital, we can much more securely and easily hold on to a humanistic truth. The truth that health is about people, not initiates. That what counts is what actually *works*. That only the individual knows. That this interrogative gains its definition and explanatory power from "within". That defining "founding values" or national symbolism—these the flags of the NHS—overlook post-modern realities and digital scope. Of course, people subscribe simultaneously to several themes: better care for oneself, for people in a similar condition, and for the community as a whole. Some seek empowerment over each category of involvement. And, in a plural society, ethnic and cultural views differ. But for most, illness is lonely; it is the quality of personal life which impacts most. Individuals have to cope. They should have the power to assess treatments in advance in terms of quality of life outcomes. Digital technology will ask uncomfortable questions—both of patients, of doctors, and of politics.

In the NHS—as in all cultural constructs—language matters. Language is fossilised metaphor. The use of words like "empowerment", "knowledge", "expertise", "partnership", and "consultation", "patient", "disease", "illness" need to be unpacked. This is to open out their composition, structure and origin. This is to ask us to notice, as Wittgenstein says, "what we say when", and the ways in which language reflects the content of practice. That is, who is the "expert"? What do we mean by "health"? And by "illness" and "disease"? These words are assumptions about reality. They embody confining cultural expectations. They do not name facts, but intentions and beliefs. They are predictive labels, in the *cultural act* of inventing spaces to occupy. They control expectations. They are about possession and dispossession and point of view. They offer pinchbeck partnerships. They give cultural circulation to specific ideas and strategies about what it is to "know" and to "be". Notably, about who has which power and knowledge to exercise and in which space. Notably, to define what we mean by "health", and who is to direct whom. This is to examine highly structured anticipations embedded in training and socialisation, and in usually unchallenged entities. These notions curtail self-reflection, self-understanding, self-responsibility, and self-empowerment. These definitions of knowledge limit us as individuals in experiencing ourselves. And they thus limit what the individual and the NHS can hope to achieve. Yet each of us alone recognises that what matters is our "inside"—not only our physical organs, but our psychology, our expectations, our values. This knowledge must become both holistic and transparent *to us*, guiding choices to be made in our *own* terms. Medicine needs to recognise and incorporate quality of life, which only patients can judge for themselves. Prior assessment about standard treatment options and their implications must be built into consent, choice, and evidence based practice. And so in recognition we must invest in collecting and processing this knowledge, once it has been re-defined and re-positioned. This is a very different approach to that which "grants" a person "rights".

The word "empowerment" has been an orphan. *Chambers Dictionary* (1994) offers a definition. "Empowerment: the giving to individuals of power to take decisions in matters relating to themselves, esp. (in an organisation) in relation to self-development." Empowerment has latterly (and unpersuasively) been re-phrased by the NHS—the insider politics are revealing—so that it incorporates neither sanction nor devices to compel. "Empowerment" has taken on the restrictive guise of (necessarily unequal) "partnership". The NHS has struggled "since Tuesday was a week" (in the phrase of a classic outsider, J. M. Synge) to give empowerment shape and meaning.[11] It has not given this priority. Rather, it has hesitated to invite increased demands. It *is* a genuine difficulty how to achieve a user-led service and at what cost. Yet the impact of multi-media interactive technology is going to be a massive challenge to resolve these difficulties, in favour of listening to patients. Empowerment looks likely to accost the system compellingly and intrusively. Information, judgments, narrative experience, comparative (and international) results will be reported by consumers to others. Certainly, too, it is going to cost the system money. There will, in my view, be net gains, for individual patients, for health status, for a society of openness, choice and self reflective responsibility.

There is here another very large public policy issue—as Perri 6, Research Director of Demos, has pointed out.[12] To what degree can the NHS and the nation deliver a maximum scenario of patient power on a routine basis over a large range of purposes? To what extent is a user-focused NHS organisationally plausible, coherently feasible, and sustainable? There may be a gain to democracy and citizenship as a result of a user-focused NHS, but what is the nature of the costs and challenges? Perri 6 suggests that these are unknown, that the contradictions are immense, that there are many collective action dilemmas, that the wish of individuals to be involved in either strategic or specific decisions is uneven. Another difficulty is that governments may seek to give legitimacy to rationing decisions which they lack the political capital to endorse alone. A further problem is the impact of such complexities as religious beliefs and bio-ethics, as well as the risks of demand for (further) "ineffective" care. On this general view, it may ultimately be necessary to negotiate a more modest scenario, in which pressure groups forcefully press an interest in rationing debates, allied to strengthened individual advocacy. This may give a welcomed gain at an acceptable cost. There is, of course, the acknowledged difficulty that these initiatives may readily be absorbed, that compelling change may only be delivered if we move beyond a modest scenario, with a different orientation, assumptions, preferences, and ways of opening our letter-boxes.[13] The important work at Demos emphasises that alternative scenarios must be costed, discussed, and addressed. But the costs are not merely economic; there are many aspects on which a value must be placed, including what notion of society is being chosen, the value of actions based on ethical commitments and on self-directed, voluntary co-operation in civic society. Digital innovations will help drive this analysis. For the moment, tempted by a maximalist scenario, I put my comfort in Sidney Webb, who (though a technocrat) somewhere remarked to a critic, that "Your arguments lead to my conclusions". For the additional costs may be requisite, with major net health care benefits. New technologies ask the unasked questions about these overlooked cultural deficits. There are other reasons to seek the empowered, involved, understanding, self-reflective, self-responsible individual. Such an invoice would notice our psycho-social interiors and quality of life issues; new perceptions of personal responsibility rooted in self-reflection, and the urgent imperatives of chronic care management. These all coincide. Greater understanding of the determinants of health status suggest the importance of self-esteem, coping strategies and their impact on the immune system. Together, these observations seem likely to be so compelling that the costs of significant and urgent change will need to be borne. Empowerment and its possible gains over policy and over personal service will not be delivered by a politicised emphasis on supply-side stability nor by polished processes. For what is required is a complete re-orientation of the system focused on the consumer. With a philosophical conviction that we can expect more from ourselves. Focused on "wants", not "needs". Focused on the networked inter-action of multi-media digital innovation which makes up the deficits, which public policy may not be able to halt. This view asks for a philosophy of technology and a technology for choice, underpinned by a belief in the special and transforming powers of choice itself, as Isaiah Berlin and before him Hayek have argued.[14]

This is, of course, to argue from a particular point of view about fundamentals. This is the view, anchored in liberalism, that all that is done must track back from the objective of what it is that "works" for the individual, who owns the body. It is this valley view which must engage all, with the passion and skill to serve and succeed. The requirement is not merely to buff particles, to fix pieces. To re-engineer is no longer divine; this approach has reached its institutional and political limits. Supply-side reform alone has, indeed, resulted, as one commentator has said, in a health care system which is "leaner, more efficient, with exhausted providers and dissatisfied customers".[15] There is an alternative, with which we are concerned here. One which takes account of a more optimistic belief about the transforming powers of choice and liberty. This alternative is to enable the health care system to re-orientate itself, by a creative focus on learning, listening, accessing the special knowledge that patients alone have—even if they do not always appreciate what they know. This will change focus, roles, components, the whole mind-set of the system. The justifications are societal and rooted, too, in the grounds of what will determine better health. This will retire from the zenith those self-evidently ineffective and clumsy, devices—"planning" and "strategy"—which have been poor predictors of future changes. This argument advances a view which works backwards from another frame of mind. For (as one literary critic, Sue Roe, has said in a different context) the task is "to embark on the painful, frustrating, sometimes excruciating business of discerning the difference, between looking and really paying attention—*really*—looking". That is, for management "to look in a mirror of their own making, to see themselves all written backwards".[16] Digital innovation will enable and require this reflection. Management will be unable to stand distant and storklike, quiet and unaware.

An individual could have five kinds of knowledge:

1. Diagnostic: What's wrong with me? And what works? What are the options, the risks, the benefits; and the alternatives and their risks and benefits?
2. Tactical: Who offers which therapies, and who is good at them? Who says so, and where is the evidence for me to see? Who designed this evidence, and to which purposes?
3. Access: Can I get it? How?
4. Narrative: What is the narrative experience of other patients like me, of this treatment, this hospital, this doctor?
5. Personal: Who am I? Information as knowledge which arises from the individual's own attempt to make sense of self and of illness and disease, as each of us learns to trust and live with our own instincts, feelings, and illnesses. Self-knowledge, self-reflection, self-responsibility.

To discover good answers, patient empowerment—digital empowerment—seems likely to be a key driver for a different NHS in a different "New Jerusalem". The NHS, of course, maintains its high "social capital" despite offering fewer rights and choices than in many other systems. This contrast is, however, becoming transparent on the Internet. The NHS—which has still to successfully computerise such a basic as NHS personal numbers—remains exempt from an open, efficient, vigorous market, even within the expected regulation of any health market. It is a system, too, which hides crucial data on who does what and how well. Yet interactive multi-media networks—what Toffler called "that great, growling engine of change, technology"—now drives "the roaring current of change". Making deficits and choices explicit to patients, and policies, priorities and health politics open to challenge.[17]

There are startling technical changes and patient opportunities. There are swift advances across every fixed technical boundary. In digital processing power and speed, in fibre-optic technology, in advanced compression and encoding, in transmission breadth and quality, in inter-activity, in the evolution of computers towards multi-media desk-top domestic and mobile applications, in the realisation of computers that can be voice-driven and which "learn" you. Now, too, agreed international standards ensure that networks are compatible and connected. This offers basic connectivity, common gateways and interfaces, scaleability—all of which will accommodate growing usage, mobility, and mass access at low prices. The key component is digital. Delivery is without boundaries. Bandwidth is facilitating multi-media inter-active quality transmissions. Multi-media is rapidly becoming the technology of choice. The key is that it is interactive, and personal. Global public access is customizing services, and penetrating honeycombed obscurity and opacity.

Medicine and health care is both existential and societal. Digital innovation is changing the possible answers to the two rugged questions: "who am I?", and "what is the system to be?" It is, crucially, about "who am I?". And, as we unfold genomics, animal re-design, genetic screening and therapy programmes to correct "flaws" and increase life-expectancy, it may even become, perhaps, who was I *designed* to be.[18]

Technologies are, however, not merely instrumental. They embody assumptions and values. Technology can help articulate a different health system. Yet choices about technologies are choices about politics, since technical life has political substance. This needs to be considered with caution. For technologies are not merely about what Jacques Ellul calls "la technique". These may or may not increase participatory democracy, decentralized political control, social equality, and reduce concentrations of power. But it is these issues which are at the heart of people's lives and relationships, and of our system of government. Yet such ideas, linked to ideas about openness, are not well developed in the NHS, because they represent fundamental challenges, especially to centralised controls. Discussions of technology and "empowerment" (and of other "democratic" innovations in localities) should ask whether the experience of health care can be something other than an experience of hierarchy and controls. Whether questions about health care can satisfactorily be defined as issues of efficiency. And what the benefits will be if we take seriously what patients tell, in their letters, their complaints, their comments, their reports, and in the unsaid, in the silent spaces between the words. These perspectives offer a basis for a public opinion, which, as David Green has said, will be "a genuinely independent sphere of thought", in which there is "a public but not political domain of duties to care".[19] These questions pose fundamentals about central or local control, legitimacy, diversity, decision-making, whose answers will be embodied technologically. These questions make it clear that it is not sufficient for the individual merely to be the target for an improved service. The issue is whether technology can help articulate a different health system within a liberal view of an open, democratic society.

What matters most is the individual's position relative to the accomplishment of their legitimate personal goals, and to social institutions. As Langdon Winner has stressed: "A primary source of legitimacy for many of the systems that form the heart of the technological society was that consumption was still centered in the individual. Any notion that ordinary people might want to have control over production or have a say in decisions beyond those of the immediate enjoyment of goods and services seemed out of the question."[20] As multi-media develop, there remains the very significant difficulty of whether or not individuals will become more or less dependent on large and complex systems which may remain, in practice, beyond their power to influence.

Any significant attempt to empower patients requires the decentralising of major political and economic institutions, and also a change in the relative position of the individual. This would need to be accomplished on different terms to the NHS reforms, which reflect centralised models and mind-sets. It would also require changes in how technologies are managed. This would be a drastic undertaking which is not captured or reflected in notions of "partnership" within a centralised structure. It would involve changes in public roles, public rules, institutions, and the relations of government—including its symbiosis with veto organisations which bargain for benefits, using economic power to exert political power. There will clearly be the recurrent need to re-negotiate a new balance of competing interests and ideals in the political marketplace, as necessary political choices have to be faced amongst competing and conflicting choices. If we are to take "empowerment" seriously, we need to clarify our goals, the required structure of institutional authority, the ends to guide us, our social ideals. We need to be clear that information is not necessarily knowledge, and that neither necessarily constitute power for educated judgment and effective individual action. "Information", and "knowledge", indeed, are but two conditions which affect the phenomenon of power. Vital is the further expectation that people are capable of self-reflective responsibility.

It is important not to be ahistorical. Historically, technology has strategically tended towards fewer centres where action is initiated and control is exercised. The multi-media revolution will not necessarily empower the individual. If new technology is not merely to benefit the already powerful then institutions mediating that power are essential. There is an issue here about the accessibility and number of local centres of decision-making, and of how these can change the power of the individual relative to government and public administration. It remains to be seen if new multi-media technology can overcome the capacity and resistance of vested interests, to alter the norms of centralised technologies, and to re-create what Peter Kropotkin (for example) would have recognised as small scale, directly democratic and widely dispersed centres of authority. This is partly an issue of local government, partly of individual exertion. It is not only an issue of information. Nor are dispersed contact points in themselves necessarily equivalent to dispersed power and autonomy. We need to search new technologies, for opportunities and for snares; we need to discipline technology in terms of social ends. What cultural philosophers have considered since Aristotle will not necessarily be achieved by technology. Langdon Winner states this clearly: "The important task becomes, therefore, not that of studying the "effects" and "impacts" of technical change, but one of evaluating the material and social infrastructures specific technologies create for our life's activity. We should try to imagine and seek to build technical regimes compatible with freedom, social, justice, and other key political ends."[21]

The digital horse is galloping up-country. It is steadily personalising and customising services, bringing greater access, and identifying vacuums where information should be but isn't. It is bringing creative and practical connections which will enable all to take part in the personal search of society, soul, silhouette, scalpel, and sensibilia. Our politics must empower these changes. Our words, as often used to conceal as to reveal, need to be articulate where they are often merely fluent.

Epic and intimate: *Les Enfants du Paradis*. Channel, content, and culture

The individual seeks two things from the NHS. These are the narrative choices posed by Marcel Carné's *Les Enfants du Paradis*:

epic, and intimate. Epic: the comfort and re-assurance of knowing that guaranteed service is there when wanted. Intimate: to be treated as a person, perceived as an individual. To be offered specific, relevant, timely, safe, kind care. Epic, as a socially integrating solace. Intimate, for personal survival and for coping with one's own present and future. Care which delivers *both* survival on acceptable terms and a quality of life apt for the individual. With both thought about openly in advance, on the terms and in the terms of the individual's values. In the personal context, the great gain will be twofold. First, that health care is not necesssarily to be experienced as a system of hierarchy and control. Second, that "ordinary" people learn the tough questions to ask, and require answers which work for them, and in a vocabulary and language that is meaningful to them. There will, too, be a cumulative effect on provision for future carers, who will themselves seek amendments. Such changes may be the only way to enhance elusive social sanction for change, by opening out reality. They will identify honestly those implicit dilemmas of moral and practical choice between necessarily irreconcilable hopes. Clearly, the questions of empowerment over general public health issues are different from empowerment over what actually happens to an individual. For "I" am not a probability but a person. This is in part about the methodology of consultation, whether or not user involvement is to be collective or individual. There are here many complexities about how current, past and likely future users relate to "strategy". These too may be assisted by direct electronic debate to democratise decision-making by local agencies. There are issues here of how credible such de-centralisation will be, and of how the individual deals with the system and whether or not it can focus on the individual, and see the individual in ways which are "written backwards".

The challenges of public and personal, or epic and intimate, in some sense coincide. It is a real question as to whether or not there is a public interest which cannot be met by an individualised process, and which is different to the aggregation of individual interests. And, if there is a gap, what is it and how could it be covered? Society needs to achieve a blend between new forms of active citizenship and of informed consumerism. People do, of course, often have mixed motives. It is not a very fine judgment to question the existing balance, processes and results. In the quandary between epic and intimate the interactive Internet will prompt the patient—Erikson's "universe of one"—to stop seeing the NHS as a "channel", and to perceive it instead as "content". They may stop seeing it in epic terms alone—as a vaguely defining national cultural asset. Instead, they will be enabled to *inspect* it in intimate terms, as a personal asset over which they will expect to exert some control. The fresh element is interactive multi-media in the comfort and trust of home. This is an innovation for piquancy. It will help people ask for care which improves survival, both in the odds quoted and in terms of their own definitions of quality of life. This is the essence of *Les Enfants du Paradis.* For it is clear that there is much more to being healthy than simply being alive.

Multi-media networks are cognitive and collaborative. They will change frames of mind, ways of seeing and believing. The parallel is with an earlier spark to literacy and understanding. This prior model of mind, the great 18th century *Encyclopedia*, suggested that new systems will not only more readily supply a certain body of accumulated (if hidden) knowledge. Like the *Encyclopedia*, it is there, as d'Alembert said in France, "pour changer la façon communé de penser"—to change the way people think.[22] This is to ponder more than merely gadgets. Clearly, improved systems matter, and there are many. For example, digital communication replaces voice communication, which does not follow the patient. In voice communication much data is lost; it is, too, unreliable and not reproducible. Digital communication offers archival data (and a basis for outcomes studies); it is transportable with patients, it enforces information rules. It offers a formidable list of innovations for rapid quality treatment, with the electronic transfer of health care information from one location to another by telemedicine, teleconsulting, telepathology, telecare in community care, telerobotic surgery. These deliver data to core sites, to the point of clinical decision-making, with archival permanence, replication and control including live-image updates and networking access. This gives high-speed community access, productivity gains, distant supervision of work at multiple sites, global off-site consultation, improved emergency room coverage, the integration of all health care tools, information and imagery. There is now multi-media referral and response, CD ROM medical reference, distance learning, virtual modelling and visualisation, gizmos in the blood-stream, electron microscopes and the Scanning Tunnelling Microscope, implants computing internal change, heartbeat monitoring and diagnosis on-line, touch-screen patient information, even the prospect of DNA as a "molecular computer". There are now telephone systems allowing the deaf to "talk" in a foreign language, releasing them from inhibition and disability. There is computer cornea measurement, genetic research, robotic distant surgery, on-line organ donor services. Vital as these are, they are not themselves a cultural dictionary. Instead, to select a transparent 19th century image of achievement, what is wanted is the Crystal Palace of cultural transformation which these devices will facilitate.

Beneficially, the language of the Internet is English. However, these will not be easy changes to finesse, especially within and between the professions and between people and professionals. Much of this reflection in the mirror will be a profound cultural shock. But this is a further evolutionary jump. Here, we are no different from our great grandfathers, Darwin's contemporaries, who saw the ape staring at them in the mirror. T. H. Huxley said then: "Brought face to face with these blurred copies of himself, the least thoughtful of men is conscious of a certain shock, due perhaps, not so much to disgust at the aspect of what looks like an insulting caricature, as to the awakening of a sudden and profound mistrust of time-honoured theories and strongly-rooted prejudices regarding his own position in nature, and his relations to the under-world of life."[23]

It is necessary to attempt to understand at the deepest levels what these cultural changes may involve. Central, of course, is the issue of what humans believe about themselves—their character, their potentials, their sense of identity, their "human" nature, the sources of social-bonding, what do we mean by "freedom". On the view taken there depends an idea about the purpose of social institutions and the philosophy of technology and of medicine. Our context is that the economic models of health care are about to change significantly. So, too, will the political marketplace within which care is delivered. The one is a consequence of the other. State health providers have so far avoided the product "branding", niche-marketing, content-creation and service provision which will become necessary in a virtual marketplace of diversified demand. There is much superficial marketing, yet state health authorities have been well-organised in a symbiotic relationship with governments and with veto-organisations. By contrast, consumers of State health provision have been distributed and weak.[24]

Economic analysts of the global digital changes have predicted a struggle: "Monopolies or oligopolies of knowledge have been built up . . . [to support] forces chiefly on the defensive, but improved technology has strengthened the position of forces on the offensive and compelled realignments favouring the vernacular."[25] Being digital, the passive patient will be passé. So a Personal Computer (PC) is a small screen for "big sky" issues. For interactive, networked multi-media enable the individual to consider, to ask, and to be much more pressing for answers. It invites questions: who is out there? What is important is being able to find them: the search and find potential is huge. What is out there? how do I know this treatment, this outcome, this doctor is what I want? how do I know you are any good? Here is the uncaptured and essential narrative: what do the stories of other people have to tell me?

It looks as if "life on the Net" will become the mainstream of everyday life. And that it will be about information and community—and about changed concepts of community. The networked computer is a window into a three-dimensional world. It opens many dimensions, including those within the individual. It seems that people will be able to work with an object, a concept, or a business process, in a natural and intuitive way. Triumphalist advocates urge that the machine will not be in the way, but become the way. That is, the natural first point of call by which people achieve insights into complex and personal problems. Thus, interactive networks remove the limitations of geography, and replace them with availability. Hypertext removes the limitations of the printed page. "Digital living" in part removes the necessity of being in a specific place at a specific time. CD ROM and the World Wide Web (WWW) will bring into the home networked information services.[26]

Computers redesign intelligence. They now filter, sort, prioritise and manage multi-media on our behalf. They act as search-agents, editors and selectors of information. They ask us questions about ourselves. We will expect good information on everything. It will not be tolerable for this merely to encompass trivial applications. It will not be accepted that it should exclude that which matters most, our health. As a direct consequence, computers will dilute the diagnostic monopoly of doctors, just as they improve consultation at a distance. They will enable the individual to re-assess the rationality of each component. Here is the unfulfilled potential for empowerment since information will be universally accessible, and the demand for missing information ineluctable. Information will be withdrawn both from data banks, and as "knowledge" from "within". As cost and access barriers are removed professional defences will alter, since these are necessarily historical. It will not be possible for people to do their jobs without good information. The filtering and design of information will be a design issue for the user, not merely for the projector. New content, new attitudes, new advocacy to support its use will all change relationships. The change is irrevocable, and exponential. "Why not?" will be the patient's daily question.

This will have a major impact on authority, and on rationing and on service provision. It will ask questions about the acceptability of services and how their qualities are defined. Networked information will *personalise* the rationing dilemma. This debate will cease to be wholly about equity—always provided the moral requirement for a good, effective, basic minimum is guaranteed by regulation. The debate will instead be about customised services, and about what the individual is prepared to fund for themselves in addition to a tax-based common minimum. Networking will shift the thresholds people will accept and those burdens people will accept. It will demonstrate that the individual has to do the rationing for themselves. This itself is empowering, since it will be up to the individual to make the trade-offs, to balance the use of expensive new technologies in return for other access and lower prices, to limit themselves, to find out about quality, to re-distribute personal resources, to express cost-conscious choices, to seek acceptable service. It looks as if you cannot have empowerment without personalising the rationing dilemma. This will inevitably query the financial structure basic to the NHS. It will prompt insured care-plans, initially based on state taxation funds, between the individual and the GP, between the individual and the private provider, as well as top-up insurance and ordinary top-up payments out of current cash.

So one cobwebby reference point is "rationing". Rationing will no longer be able to be managed by denial and delay. Computing, patient values and informed health care will converge. The rationing criteria will become personal. Explicitness will challenge legitimacy. It will not remain possible to ration on the grounds of "effectiveness", nor on the grounds of probability, which is necessarily uncertain. The individual will wish to decide what is acceptable to them. The individual will wish to decide what "works" for them, since these are genuinely personal and not impersonally technical questions. The view to be heard is that of both the patient and of the citizen—these may be different mind-sets but the clarification of this issue will prompt basic questions about health financing. This will follow as patients more independently seek to change the ways in which professionals hear them, and think about them and with them. The problems of "voice", "exit" and sanction are, of course, inextricably entwined with assumptions about roles, "expertise", "knowledge" and with issues of finance.

Multi-media will necessitate the re-orientation of the entire system pivoted on personalised, customised services, by contrast to non-discriminatory mass-access. It will affect patients' know-how, and their attitudes to what they know intuitively but which the system does not access. It will change the ability of providers to attract and to manage capital resources; the legitimacy and accountability of "proxy agents" and purchasers of health care; roles and relationships, processes and government. Empowerment, whatever the territory afforded or enabled, can itself only become real—for patients and for staff—if linked to empowering devices for sanction, notably the compelling power of money. This is not only the language of business. It is the language of morality, with its emphasis on well-being. It is the language and the insight of the novelist, too, if we are to release feelings, wishes, preferences, and coping strategies to impact on what determines health, and to enhance participation in common institutions.[27]

Great British novelists have presented doctors to us—Charles Dickens, George Eliot, Jane Austen. They have agreed, too, that we are a deeply secretive people. A century or more later, we still hide in "mass" society. Mystery, too, has been an essence of our reality. Indeed, mystery was an early collective noun for doctors.[28] Yet the utility of this frame of mind is coming to its end. We have held too exclusively to the bio-medical model. We have doubted too long the value of listening to our own instincts. We have given too little thought to how to listen, nor have we noticed that we do not (in Sue Roe's terms) *really* do it. We have reserved to novelists and poets the narrative benefits of the individual experience of others, and, instead, held as a compass to "scientific", targeted reason, to scientific rationality. We can now see how damaging this has been. We need to respect the utility of narrative from patients and to empower it. New technology offers this. We need Jane

Austen's echoing framework for what she says in *Northanger Abbey*: "Oh! it is only a novel! . . . or, in short, only some work in which the greatest powers of the mind are displayed, in which the most thorough knowledge of human nature, the happiest delineation of its varieties, the liveliest effusions of wit and humour, are conveyed to the world in the best chosen language."[29]

Charles Babbage was twenty seven when that was published, just posthumously, in 1818, although his "Difference Engine" had not intruded upon Chawton and its mysteries of the heart. Yet, nearly two centuries later, interactive multi-media is bringing these very qualities—discrimination, trust in intuitive feelings, faith in narrative experience, commitment to quality of life in outcomes—into policy focus. It is, too, shifting professional views of patient capacities, as education and interactive-media combine to encourage the self-responsible service-user essential to health care re-definition and improvement. This offers a new socialisation for medicine, by people. To this felicity and consolation we have to credit electricity, grains of sand and glass-fibres. And, too, to greater understanding of the determinants of health. In particular, the role of self-esteem, its impact on immune systems, and the distinction between "disease" (scientific, objective) and "illness" (personal, lonely).[30] We know—from the studies of McKeown, Evans, Sagan, Marmot, the McKinlays—that changes in the nature of medical care *systems* have limited impacts, since these systems are not the major determinants of health.[31] Many conventional explanations about why some people are healthier than others are wrong or incomplete. Yet massive investment continues to go into "planned" health care systems, possibly mistakenly or incoherently. The availability or absence of curative services does not seem to explain observed differences among the health of populations. "Health care" and "health" are not synonymous. We need to find the other *initiating* forces and causes of good health as Evans argues. Self-esteem, empowerment, future orientation, perceived personal status, effective personal coping strategies seem vital, seem to impact on the immune system, and should be supported by innovation. Here, technical innovation will innovate perceptions.

There are organisational consequences. One need is for interpretative, intuitive leaders with flair and creativity, who want good service for patients and understand that the key to effective management is the notion of "open systems", as Peter Senge has taught.[32] Successful managements have changed strategy, to work in open systems, to release the knowledge of patients and the skills of staff. As Nicholas Negroponte says: "In an open system we compete with our imagination, not with a lock and key".[33] An open system supports a wider variety of choice for the consumer, and a nimble commercial sector capable of rapid change and growth. It could put transparent public service into the public domain, and help to change definitions of public values. Open systems are designed to ensure services accessible to all. The future for health systems is open-architecture. The past (which William Faulkner says is not dead, it is not even past) is local and closed monopoly. Such past but surviving structures will be unable to deny the power of networked communications. These, as Negroponte points out, are decentralising, harmonising, globalising, and empowering. Open systems enable decentralised structures; the political marketplace disables them. Yet a highly interconnected and decentralised structure will be more resilient, more inventive, more coherent. It will survive through adaptability. The future of health systems is the networked interface between distributed agencies and organisations. An open system, and one in which skilled and creative doctors—no enfants—will almost certainly take command. But in a new context set by patients.

No country called Technopolis: Cares, categories and criteria

The Internet is both model and metaphor. Yet before we agree that multi-media computer networks must inexorably change everything—and that "progress" is inevitable—let us pause. Before we assume positive advance, net gain, and cultural enrichment, we need to be sure about our philosophy of technology. For our philosophy of the individual is embedded within it. Langdon Winner, ten years ago, sought to articulate the case for a political philosophy of technology. He set out, in a mere one hundred and twenty nine words, those immensities of which we are now all suddenly aware of in our lives. These immensities are again altering the ways we live, relate to one another, and experience the world and ourselves.

Winner says: "The map of the world shows no country called Technopolis, yet in many ways we are already its citizens. If one observes how thoroughly our lives are shaped by interconnected systems of modern technology, how strongly we feel their influence, respect their authority, and participate in their workings, one begins to understand that, like it or not, we have become members of a new order in human history. To an ever-increasing extent, this order of things transcends national boundaries to create roles and relationships grounded in vast, complex instrumentalities of industrial production, electronic communications, transportation, agribusiness, medicine, and warfare. Observing the structures and processes of these vast systems, one begins to comprehend a distinctively modern form of power, the foundations of a technopolitan culture."[34]

Certainly, the political theory of the public institutions of a learning and multi-media information society need debate. We do not have this yet, as Peter Drucker reminds us.[35] As we consider these issues, a philosophy of technology needs to fit with the liberal philosophy which is as much about responsibilities as it is about "rights". David Green—seeking a viable, non-political alternative to state welfare, in an un-politicised community—has argued that morality and civilisation can survive only in a society where individuals live in the true sense together —where they accept responsibility both for their own lives and for the lives of others closely tied to them, through bonds of common purpose and affection—as in families, friendships and small voluntary or jointly-owned enterprises. In the face of the overwhelming power of the state individuals have no sense of control over their own existencies. The true purpose of government, instead, is to reinforce personal moral relationships, to reinforce those interpersonal institutions which arise from individual choice and individual effort. Responsibility cannot be "delivered" or commanded. Responsibility is a cultural characteristic of an economic structure. it is not "deliverable" either by paternalism or leadership. It derives instead from informed reflective duty and personal conduct which is self-directed. It is behaviour rooted in ownership, in private property rights, in individual rewards for good stewardship. That is, in the thought, knowledge and responsibility which is integral to living, part of which is the penalties for negligence which individual's experience in all other areas of living. The process of responsible living is market-based since that is where individual judgments matter, and where competing provision can be judged against its own claims to be efficient, effective, and faithful; where its claims are identifiable, measurable, accountable and judged against individual preference and expectation.[36]

If a patient has a responsibility to the system, it is to co-operate in a diagnosis; thereafter, it is for the individual to decide whether or not to accept a treatment. Certainly, professional advice should be offered, and welcomed, which is also to recognise that doctors are moral agents. The difficulty is with insistence, with the absence of non-directional advice, and with traditional paternalism. In a free society, "choice", like Canis Major, should be the brightest star in all the heavens. The results would include incentives for responsibility, which derives not from paternalism and command but from self-knowing. This is the context for the computer, within the imperatives of modern health care.

Langdon Winner saw that we create artificial realities which reconstruct the on-going conditions of human existence. He saw that these were about new connections, and newly uncovered cultural structures, about who we want to be, how we think about our own faculties and activities, and what kind of a world we want to live in. This asks—in a long tradition of ambivalence about the man–machine syndrome and the terrified allure of symbiosis—whether, and if so how, we can work with multi-media to negotiate change to set out a framework in which we are persistently human.

The basic task for a philosophy of technology is to examine critically the nature and significance of artificial aids to human activity. This is not merely a question of focusing on "content" rather than "carriage", as a corrective to much triumphalist writing, necessary as that is. It is a question of the subtle relationships between both. Winner has clarified this: "the important question about technology becomes, As we 'make things work', what kind of world are we making?" We need to pay attention not only to the making of physical instruments and processes, but also to the production of psychological, social, and political conditions as a part of significant technical change. Are we going to design and build circumstances that enlarge our possibilities for growth in human freedom, sociability, intelligence, creativity, and self-government—within which health care systems are subsumed. Or are we headed in an altogether different direction, where health care will inevitably be experienced as hierarchy and control?

This discussion offers the idea that technical things have political qualities. These are non-trivial questions, asked notably by Lewis Mumford, Jacques Ellul and Herbert Marcuse—and more recently by Bruce Mazlish, Jerry Mander, Theodore Roszak, Clifford Stoll, and Stephen Talbott. These cultural critics ask fundamental questions about which ideas, attitudes, behaviours, about which institutions, professions and organisations have generally benefited most from new technologies. About whether computers enable governments to assist or resist de-centralisation, whether they dangerously re-define education, how a computer mono-culture impacts on "primitive" societies, about what a world-wide electronic mono-culture is destroying as well as creating.[37]

Winner states that "judgment, action, and change are ultimately products of history."[38] There is so much change going on—such a cornucopia of information, advertisement, euphoric boostering, that it is easy to focus on the narrow view of which new device serves which need, which is cost-effective, which is convenient, which is styled right for you. We see here the unreflective assumption that technological change is a cause from which to follow inevitable effects. Thus the role of humans is to adapt to what is next, rather than to notice and consider dilemmas and to make decisions about them. At first sight, then it looks as if the pace of technological change and interconnectedness has already succeeded in constructing a cultural reality which is principally a technical system. One in which human beings are individually subsumed in social roles and relationships whose pace and shape is deeply influenced by technology. In such a system it is implied that in our lives "life" will be difficult without the technology. Yet the big-sky issues remain the broad ones of "meaning", and of using the technology for democracy and openness, to correct the assymetrics of information, power and direction. We need clarity about what multi-media means for moral and social life, for relationships, for the quality of life. Techniques and systems are not our purpose, they are procedures to purposes. Nor should we focus on the momentum of change itself, fast as is its pace, or necessarily be gripped by the idea of "progress".

The real question is not just that technologies are aids to human activity. As Winner says: "Individual habits, perceptions, concepts of self, ideas of space and time, social relationships, and moral and political boundaries have all been powerfully restructured in the course of modern technological development. What is fascinating about this process is that societies involved in it have quickly altered some of the fundamental terms of human life without appearing to do so. Vast transformations in the structure of our common world have been undertaken with little attention to what those alterations mean."[39]

Technical forms are implicated in the basic patterns and problems of our culture. These developments have changed our material life; our ways of relating to one another. They have even shaped our sense of what it is to be a human being. This is seen in the language of "networking", "interface", "feedback". We compare our minds to the operations of a computer. Our understanding of technological devices has merged with our instinctive understandings of one another and of ourselves. We are now being shaped in mind, pace, and skills by the new multi-media led by computers. And, as in the past, technology will be instrumental in social movements seeking to transform social relations. Thus, through computers, the hope of the electronic democracy, the computer as de-centralising instrument for change, the promise of the information age providing a more egalitarian society.

And so the problem of new multi-media and health is not merely an issue about the sociology of improvement. Nor only about how providers will interlock, and network. It offers a discussion of what Winner calls "a richer set of cares, categories, and criteria." It asks for us to apply a wider range of concepts concerning "knowledge", "expertise" and individual worth. This asks the question of how can the computer change our politics, and empower the individual within themselves, to what wider social as well as health care purposes. Technologies can follow a number of different paths, depending on the assumptions and interests of those who develop and support them. In medicine, as Edward Tenner argues, the retreat from intensity would imply a movement away from the prerogatives of professional power, of political endorsement of that power and of the intensities of volume, away from acute medicine to preventative medicine, and towards investment in support systems—mainly social systems—in the home. And, of course, technologies can impact on patient empowerment to assist understanding in self-reliant modes of being.

The tools of change are intellectual, as well as electronic. But they are not in themselves solutions. We should recognise, too, that our need is not that of reverse-adaptation, in which life is re-shaped to fit the technical means available. Rather, it is to shape the technical apparatus for moral ends. Here, in the words of T. S. Eliot, "the first condition of right thought is right sensation."[40]

The Internet as infrastructure: A research laboratory for public policy

The Internet and the World Wide Web is an *infra-structure*, not a solution.

It offers the expectation that better quality care and individual empowerment will be delivered. It is a research laboratory for public policy. It will increase the pressures on the NHS, and focus attention on demand-side issues and deficits which remain unaddressed. These pressures will beguile those questions of philosophy and values which remain unanalysed. Most essentially, interactive multi-media will enable the individual to discriminate risk, to be linked to others, to find out who and what is "out there" and what is "in here". The revolution in information will show, too, that information is both missing and yet not the only necessity. Additional devices for empowered leverage will be wanted if the technology is to fulfil its potential for improved care by greater choice, empowerment, and liberty (within which responsibility is not only subsumed, but embedded).

It is necessary to find devices which will complement information and evidence, which will accommodate stories, which help to generate them, which will provide incentives—not only financial—to supply it. That is, a structure of understanding and of behavioral incentives for consumer-led decision-making. One which offers good entrances and easier exits within agreed boundaries, and which are compatible with the revising missions of professionals, patients and politicians. There need to be personal advantages to signing-up. The costs will also have to be borne.

The tools of change are thus intuitive and narrational, intellectual, political, technical. Holding hands with Langdon Winner, take technical. We are now seeing quite startling global technical innovations. Most fundamentally, too, these are coming into the home, bringing an enormous range, depth and detail of information. For the consumer, as for the doctor, the importance of memory and of "library skills" will diminish. Information will be current, and universal. It will not be a commodity, but an instrument. Medical students, too, will discover a different education, and perhaps a changed socialisation. The affordably omni-present PC-TV or Networked Computer will rapidly become the most familiar, most-utilised, perhaps most-trusted of *domestic* instruments. It will also network all the others, as a communications medium and tool. It will be inclusive on a class basis, too, like the satellite dish which strongly appealed to members of classes categorised as C and D. It will change discussions with medical professionals, in a new equilibrium. Marshall Marinker noted first in his 1980 Oration to the Reading Pathological Society all of these likely shifts. He said: "values which we attach to aspects of character, personality and problem-solving in the clinician may change. Skills in empathy, in forming and using a therapeutic relationship, in thinking divergently over large and changing aspects of the patient's life, may become the hallmark of what patient and doctor value most."[41]

Digitalisation of all media and all networks will allow all audio and video content to be used, re-used, and re-arranged at will. In important respects there is the potential for the user to be in control; to be both *publisher* and expert; to express expectations with new power and confidence; to expect customisation of service and differentiation by the functioning of interactive-markets in which organisations change fundamentally. Providers will be expected to deliver full video and audio to the individual desktop, and not merely words to the public library reference dust. This will be a new relationship between consumer and provider. When the PC can readily network, inexpensively, and be easily used then a global mass market will be in place. Simplification within concealed complexity is the objective. This is now being fulfilled. Prices, too, are lowered by technical innovation, volume, expectation, and competition. The PC is now combining with the TV, which the "mass market" already uses for its information source. Here, people are comfortable with "projection", which will be increasingly customised. The machine itself will ask questions, and deliver bespoke answers. There will be direct marketing to individuals on wrist watch computers which talk to PCs via infra-red links. Acorn's NetStation or network computer, proffered at £399, will plug into a standard TV and provide "viewers" simple access to the Internet. This new computing architecture is no longer based merely on the PC. It is framed by inexpensive network computers, which will now simplify use. They will have no floppy discs or hard-drives, and so no installation or up-dating problems. The NetStation is able to be upgraded online, accessing external software via the Internet. A key driver for adoption will be the lure of Virtual Reality experience, with its engaging nature and its entertainment and training potentials. Another will be the telephone. The number of people using the Internet to make telephone calls at local rates is projected to grow from 500 000 to 16 million by 1999. House design is, too, already moving to a swifter march. Homes are now being built with pre-installed high-quality, wide bandwidth networks.

The PC is not a stand-alone instrument for personal productivity. It is a networked information tool which is becoming the centre of business and personal communications via client/server systems. They are used to send faxes, e-mail, to share databases, to automate work-flow, for long-distance video-conferencing, as a strategic tool in network management and a personal tool for informing and effecting choices. People are becoming accustomed to calling up work on a PC, discussing it over the telephone, down-loading what they want (even while they sleep) to keep or work with. This is the consumer as activist and as publisher. In a digital world users can create their own publications; they need no longer be the passive recipient of information in printed form. They will, instead, proactively decide to issue information, opinion, stories of narrative experiences, and request similar material. Hypertext links and intelligent agents on the Internet will eliminate the periodicity preferred by publishers, and by NHS organisations. Data will need to be competitively current. Information will have to be as close to absolutely live as possible. The presumption will be that necessarily all information is up to date and cast in the form of intelligence which users want. The user will decide what they want, when they want it, how they want it. This viewpoint will inevitably become linked directly to spending power. If a tax-based system does not deliver change, it will be queried and amended.

The existing PC is already delivering much enhanced bandwidth to the desktop, with the simultaneous development of multi-media tools directed from the domestic PC. This is the most dynamic segment of the growing computer/multi-media market. It will re-define relationships throughout the health industry. It will do so with linked-tools which will enable the user to be very well-informed. The PC-TV/Network Computer is coming into the living room for family use as part of the family entertainment system and every story will be told, every question asked. The PC market is the centre of innovation. Video and audio editing software is now pre-installed so that users can work with interactive media from the day of purchase. Video-conferencing (and document sharing) systems now allow users to see and hear partners, anywhere on the globe. This is now cheap to use for personal tele-conferencing. PC-based tele-conferencing is going to be widespread, in addition to its use for large room-based meetings necessary for groups of health professsionals using installations set up with large screens, acoustic panels, microphones and special lighting, for "virtual workgroups" in a competitive environment requiring quick decision-making. The quality of image now shows subtle communication-clues such as body-language. Usage in medical practice will go on growing quickly, especially now that users of different systems can talk with one another compatibly. The "shared white-board" viewed by all parties enables all to view information, to add to it, and to record and print it, unconstrained by time or geography. Again, here is Negroponte's call by the digital individual: "tell me more".

Personal video-conferencing (although still not yet of high quality imaging) will increase the efficiency of medical professionals. It will also enhance the empowerment of the individual patient. These systems are no longer the preserve of large multinationals and niche markets. The introduction of international standards is freeing systems from proprietary controls, and allowing inter-operability between systems. Together with falling prices and the wider availability of high-speed digital telecom links, usage is growing rapidly. In particular, sales for systems based on desktop personal computers and computer networks (now down to £1500) are growing rapidly. By their very nature, interactive multi-media offer a discontinuity in virtually every area of life. Networked multi-media suggests that medicine will be one of a three-way relationship: you, me, and the machine. The last element will be as real and as commanding as the first. The "me" will be explored in self-directed dimensions. Interactive processes will replace existing passive processes. Information will face both ways: it will assist professionals and service users. In the interim, it will frighten politicians. It will change the culture, management, performance (and therefore ability to attract investment) of provider units. It will help make up the new deficits created by demography and medical innovation.

New technology will re-inforce story-telling between individuals. There are a host of solutions seeking problems. Intel's Internet Technology Laboratories have proposed a peer-to-peer technology called PandoraNet, which will allow every PC connected to the network to act as both the client and the server (that is, a computer linked to the network). Powerfully, this will go beyond client/server systems to network PCs. Time will be saved, complexity made invisible, data and choice indivisible. Costs will continue to fall. Information will become knowledge, as counselling keeps pace. Companies will cluster their PCs via this technology, too. For example, ServerNet combines hundreds of processors, and works at very high speeds, creating highly efficient systems. This is a response to the problem that numerous forms of electronic commerce, from electronic data interchange to global messaging, will demand more throughput than current processor and software-bound architectures can tolerate. Health care architectures will respond. As applications breakthrough to deliver voice, video, graphics, imagery at low cost the potential impact on demand and performance of distant-provision in medicine will be very significant.[42]

On the Net, in the parlour, access for all

How will everyone achieve access?

First, the PC-TV or Networked computer will be in every living room. It will succeed the satellite dish and the Bang & Olufsen suite.

Second, there will be high-street information and advisory centres, or Virtual Reality Health Councils (VRHC). The VRHC would achieve something important which Langdon Winner asks for in considering technological changes: "How well do the proposed conditions match our best sense of who we are and what we want this society to be? . . . To nurture this process would require building institutions in which the claims of technical expertise and those of a democratic citizenry would regularly meet face to face. Here the crucial deliberations would take place, revealing the substance of each person's arguments and interests."[43]

Third, technical barriers will be removed: voice recognition will let the elderly user and the computerphobic into this world. So far, there are a range of products (with names like DragonDictate, IBM's VoiceType, and Kurzweil Voice) which let you dictate text into Windows-based word-processors by using a microphone. They can handle 60–75 words a minute, and so far have limited vocabularies. IBM has 32 000 words, and room to add 2000. Kurzweil Voice, at a cost of £825, is a system with 20 000 word vocabulary, including many specialist medical and business terms, and with the capacity to add your own 30 000 words. Investment and ingenuity are resolving these difficulties and dissolving these boundaries. This technology will transfer to the mass-market PC-TV.

Together, all these changes will confront a defining issue: how to bridge the electronic divide which separates the information-rich and the information-poor to ensure that all consumers can benefit from new technology and the information it will reveal. The conversion of the TV into a networked PC-TV will do this. The VRHC will be an intermediate institution, for advice, support, counsel. It will also be the source of narrative knowledge from other people. It may itself prompt greater reliance on mutual and voluntary organisation.

Public systems are already being tested which hint at this. These are the early Brimstone's of a spring-time for information and narrative judgment. The UK's National Association of Health Authorities and Trusts (NAHAT) associated itself in June 1996 with an Internet advice channel, and the NHS Executive is launching its NHSweb and supports the Family Health Service Computer Unit.[44] These are management networks. The issue here is what is actually on the system—and whether the organisation is using the data to manage with. There is some justified suspicion of glorified menus, "image" web-pages from NHS Trusts. These are not an advance unless they give information which offers real choices and improved quality. Public kiosks with Touch-screen information guidance on treatments—if not generally on quality or patient narratives—is being piloted in a number of places. Camden & Islington Community Health Services NHS Trust has, however, launched in May 1996 IRIS, an Interactive Research and Information System with touch screens in two community outpatient clinics and a questionnaire function on *user* priorities. The Intouch with Health project in GP surgeries, begun in Cirencester in Spring 1996, offers treatment guidance. Cambridge OnLine links more than 4000 voluntary and self-help groups. The Swiss Co-Op bank has already used Intel's ProShare products to create personal conferencing kiosks; BMW is doing so to speed-up and improve the design process with component suppliers; BT proposes Touchpoint multimedia kiosks, and already has an interactive-TV trial in Ipswich and Colchester. Scotland's Highland Regional Council is providing public access kiosks in public buildings, for advice, learning and training. The National Citizens Advice Bureaux are creating a national on-line network. National Savings has a "Virtual Shop", on-line. Kodak is investigating high-street digital kiosks to process digital camera prints. The need is for mass-market investment.

Private sector initiatives include Racal Network Services offer of Quza, which gives structured, managed, secure access to internal and external Internet services. If information on public health is available in every high street it will be a fundamental change in the distribution of intelligence. Patients (probably in focus or special interest groups) will want to use it to talk to one another, and to health providers. The introduction of the PC/TV or Network computer will bring all this into every domestic environment, as individuals go on-line to the local VRHC and the international WWW and user-groups. Thus, both by the use of new technology within provider units and in the outside community, isolated consumers such as the disabled, the unregistered, and the geographically remote can participate in society more fully. Disability Net gives the disabled medical information and social support. Computers are enabling the disabled to learn spatial skills which will help them in the real world. The Royal National Institute for the Blind has an "Information Superhighways Project"—there are an estimated 20 000 blind or partially sighted people in the UK using computers, to work, play, enhance screen images, use speech synthesisers and braille keyboards. The technology now used is similar to that used in architectural design. Psychologists at Leicester University led by Dr Nigel Foreman have now succeeded in recreating an entire primary school building in 3-D virtual reality on a desktop computer to help disabled children develop navigational skills.[45]

It is fundamental to ask and answer the question of how will new technology assist the patient to ask for information on processes and procedures—this kind of care or that—and on how to challenge and discriminate? Where will be the information source on how to get the information? The Internet is putting doctors in touch with one another—"help me with this symptom"—and patients in touch with one another—"how did you get on? what therapy were you offered? would you do it again?" It is telling users about different approaches in different cultures, to explore different attitudes to patient autonomy, to disease management, financial structures, expenditure, and choice. It is changing the nature of information and shows that the job of the provider cannot be done without it. It will change delivery systems, and the profile of organisations. There are a number of clear and influential factors. Technology is now up to speed. People can get information when they need it. Many patients know where to look for information. They also know when it is not where they expect it to be. The Internet—with its incipient challenges of no censorship, no copyright, no barriers or bounds, and its challenges to privacy—has opened up global channels of communication which no government could have created, or afforded. Intangibly, national boundaries are dissolving, geography is being marginalised; tangibly, networks are evolving by means of a medium across which messages are conveyed into a space in which new communities can be formed and new business transacted. These opportunities for personal contact go beyond text retrieval, into a global but grassroots movement which is formulating what services people want and expect. Suppose you are told by your GP that you have "Squink's disease". As the use of the Internet grows, very large numbers will ask: What is it? Is there a support group? What are the possible treatments, options, risks, benefits of therapies? What are the side-effects of each alternative? How do I estimate probabilities, and my place on the distribution curve? What are my values, beliefs? What could I live with, cope with, manage? What quality of life and which ethical questions arise? The individual will go onto the Net and identify some information that is of interest, doing the research which they will discuss with health professionals and with other patients. This will frame the questions they bring to medicine. You will do this at home, or via the VRHC. You will download what you want to your own workstation. You may then send the material to a colleague, or to a contact on the Net. You will check various leads in the document, by clicking onto all other documents of interest in the field. Then you will go to search sources such as smart networks like Netscape, for articles of interest, and do full-text searches of publications. Intelligent search-agents will not wait to be asked: they will seek information on their own, having learnt the user's interests. They will be instructed to give recommendations. Search agents make networks smart about you; you do not need to be smart about networks. As you go onto the Web you become part of it, and so does what you add to it. You then link-up to local bulletin boards, and perhaps go on-line in real-time to other users. Your PC-TV will help you check quality, access complaints. It will analyze them, discover which doctor does which procedure often, and with what reported results. It will look at patient satisfaction, geographical location, where doctors are trained, and re-trained. It will emphasise that it is not cost-control but quality which makes the contribution, and drive providers into the quality quadrant. It will reveal drug treatments and other therapies. For example, an anti-emetic available to cancer patients in France, Germany or Spain to stop patients being sick but which may not be available here on the grounds of cost. This will prompt patients on the Internet to ask for it. They will say they want it before they are sick, not, as in the UK, once they are sick. What will happen, if the European Community seeks convergence on health care entitlements?[46]

Health organisations will have to re-orient themselves, to move information and understanding to the crossroads that will count: to point of sale, customer service, marketing, international networking. The social and customer architecture will change. Indeed, IT directors will become Customer Service Directors who truly throw clout, unlike their marginal position today. For the enterprise will itself be a network. Computing will be for client service, not for automation alone or for reports back to central base. This "client/server" computing will need to lead the organisation, since many users will access a wide range of information, applications, and computing resources before agreeing to any health intervention. An effective, competitive, productive enterprise will not be able to do its job unless this is its architecture. All operational support systems (customer service, investment, capacity planning, problem solving) will need to change focus on serving customer measured care and benefit.

We are talking about reality, not prediction. User-groups and health consumers are already comparing results, standards, outcomes, patient narrative reports, infection rates, what "works", before agreeing a treatment. People will increasingly access other patients and advice groups on the bulletin boards, where every consumer is a publisher who can create and send a message and contribute to a discussion group. An example is the Down's syndrome online group, one of tens of thousands in which people all over the world "talk" to each other, post messages, answer openly, or write privately by e-mail. POSNET, an HIV-specific service which originated in The Netherlands is a similar group, as is AIDS Treatment Update, now on the Web and attracting 50 times the number of hard-copy conventional readers. There are similar groups for diabetes, arthritis, shyness, obesity, cystic fibrositis, dyslexia and so on. Such groups do not eliminate the need for human interaction; they facilitate it. As one user said: "The people who post messages in the Down's Syndrome Net group are not just cheering each other up. They are working out their children's future, and they have everything to play for."[47] Internet cafes are another point of entry for those unsure. Another will be the high-street "gateway", or VRHC.

The content required is itself being defined by user groups. Content will increasingly be the added-value in Home Pages. As the "transactional value" of these systems gains reputation and status, even those who now commonly say "you tell me, doc" seem likely to wonder about the value of greater autonomy. Indeed, the success of the interactive Video programmes suggests that we have already underestimated patient wishes for autonomous choice supported by counselling.[48] There is, too, an argument here about community. Negroponte and Tapscott, for example offer the notion that the disintegrating impact of modern urban life will be off-set by multi-media interaction which will create and mould communities. Initially, by "virtual" contact, but with the potential of local and personal contact.

There is little doubt that very large numbers of individual PC users will come on-line into these systems, to speak to previous and potential patients, to take part in on-line user groups, to add their views to bulletin boards, to speak to chief executives of Trust and Health authorities about their complaints, their wishes, and their concerns. These systems will have a holistic impact on how providers organise themselves both internally and externally. Net discussions spread, cumulate, and remain on-line for access by anyone at any time. There is an issue of verifiability and of whether the information is relevant to me, and can I trust it. But facts are checkable, and second opinions are getable. Individual judgment and assessment is within our abilities. Loss of credibility can be very rapid. In addition the political game of playing one audience against another, not difficult when consumers are isolated and producers are organised, is more detectable, and damaging when caught. This is a new element in health markets, and in the political market.

A very influential innovation is already the digital agent. Negroponte likens this to a well-trained English butler, who knows the nuances and niggles of his employer, who knows about you and about external processes. The digital butler acts in the best interests of the employer, in loyalty and in solidarity. This will require people to manipulate computers less, and to be able to manipulate the external environment using what the computer discovers. This makes the digital marketplace real. It creates the active interface between the individual and the computer, and promotes interactive relationships. The computer itself—in constant contact with every other networked computer, gathering and analyzing health data on treatments, outcomes, practitioners and narrative comment by patients—will raise questions with the individual. The digital butler literally goes in search of what you want to know. It will search the Web and propose a treatment strategy; tell you what to check and who to check with; analyze and report on what you want to know, from knowing your beliefs, individual characteristics, health history, genetic inheritance, the kind of individual you are and what you value. Or, if your GP suggests that you need a hip replacement. you click onto "hips", "Dr Up-to-date", "Hip Advice Group", "St Hilda's", "National Orthopaedic Advice Line", "Patients Association" and start listening and talking. You can break down categories. Here is what you need to know about secondary infection rates, stay rates, pain management, choice of protheses, stories patients tell. This is a big jump beyond the performance league table and the 'phone-in helpline.

The computer will advise you of the availability of therapies, drugs, and the location of advisory and advocacy groups on the Net. It will prompt automatic joint-consultation of networked sources, of distant diagnostic opportunities of tele-medicine, as you sit with your medical "pilot" and discuss an action plan. The challenge for the next decade is to use multi-media opportunities to deliver quality that is recognised as such by users and in their own terms. The burden of interaction has shifted, from the user who has to struggle for information, to the provider who must get inside the clockwork of their organisation, and expose the quality working to the outside world. The good manager will be interested in the noticeable difference, because that is what the consumer wants. People don't want to be bothered with machines—they want service. The machine will bother with itself, and come up with the answers by searching the Net. Search and selection of a medical professional will be easy, and the Net will also show users the standards, procedures, and outcomes that are to be found in other parts of the globe. This will be dynamic. Local standards will be compared with international benchmarks—but, unlike the

Maryland project and other internally-focused initiatives, this will be in real-time and in real outside-life for patient-defined outcomes. It will not be difficult to do, and it will rapidly become first-nature in the home-computer market. The key relationship—the GP/Patient consultation—will be much enhanced. The time spent, the quality of that time, the roles of advocacy and partisan will be strengthened. The biographic role will be supported by interactive, live multi-media memory and analysis. Performance of professionals, access and price, patient reports and key indicators will be instantly available.

Digital markets are different in ways which move the pole. Companies' interest in patients will go digitally to market. The rules may say that pharmaceutical products cannot be advertised in particular ways. But this is an out-dated geographical idea. Once all this information is on the WWW, there will no longer be barriers to patients knowing and asking. Gorbachev lost the USSR in similar circumstances. Advertisers will go around the intermediate, the GP, directly to markets. The WWW is outside national frontiers. De-regulation and control—even without the "Bit police" or censorship—will become more complex, especially if patients are insistent on direct supply of drugs that they believe work, and which are available or cost less abroad. Patients will discover that there are no waiting lists in France, and ask why. They will discover that different drugs, which users say work, are not available to them, and ask why. They will discover that consumer health guidance is published in the USA, and ask why not here. They will ask for second opinions, interactive video guidance, Who's Who data on doctors, and better information and literature to prepare them to make their choices. They will, too, want to consider, for example, the Australian and the American view of patient autonomy, and different cultural ideas about the global marketplace. Physical constraints vanish. There are no boundaries to comparison shopping. Everything can be checked and re-checked with someone. Those with superior services, products, prices, will be visible; those without will no longer be invisible, or concealed from inspection by aggregate data. The consumer will thus become a digital-shopper—seeking the therapy which best supports the individual's wishes, and with cost-conscious choice. Each therapy centre will be linked in partnerships with experts elsewhere. No one centre will be an island; all will be linked in regular or ad hoc partnerships. Purchasers will keep track and form a rapid picture of the changing performance of providers on the issues that matter to the individual, and the issues that the medical adviser says are relevant and ought to matter most. This transparency itself will prompt the entry of new players, including those with proven multi-media skills. A future Virgin–Sony Healthcare Systems (relying on wide recognition and loyalty to their brands, and with their experience of information systems, risk assumption, billing and customer relations, and networking skills) seem plausible and probable market entrants. Markets have been re-defined by the Internet, and so have individuals. Voice recognition is next, and it will create genuine ease-of-access to machines which "know" us, learn us, and guide us. Whither NHS cost-income ratios?

The Internet offers unique and original learning opportunities and access to information. It invites full participation. It offers, too, the political opportunity to link individual deficits to the compelling power of money, for example with weighted "Virtual Vouchers" to enable those who do least well to have enhanced buying power. Community development, too, is within easy grasp—virtually, on the Net; actually, in real-time. There are, in fact, two revolutions of enormous significance. One is multi-media and digital (including nano-technology), the other is genetic. This may include DNA computers calculating 1000 times faster than existing computers, and a billion times more energy efficient. Both revolutions are culturally homogenising. The future may merge the two, into a ubiquitous and functional DNA. Immediately, multi-media interactive networks will change time and space dependencies, and individual expectations. The computer visitor will ask for it all on the Net: "Dr Livingstone, I presume?"

The Virtual Reality Health Council (VRHC) is an important opportunity for people to appraise before they access services. For we need institutions which are democratic in their assumptions and in their reach and which foster independence and responsibility and enhance individual competence. The VRHC would be a public device for *scrutiny* and *empowerment.* It would enable people to look at evidence, and ask what is it saying? Can you believe it? What are the "framing effects"? How relevant is it to my condition and situation? The VRHC will be a site for the development of critical appraisal skills. Its core job will be to discover the questions which are important to consumers, and to seek answers with them and in their language. It will not limit the questions to those which professionals think users should address, nor seek to restrict possible answers. It will help us develop an ability to gain knowledge and to act effectively with that knowledge, to turn information into "knowledge", and knowledge into power over outcome. For democracy is not based simply on open information. It depends on an optimistic view of the capability of people and their right to rule in full knowledge. The VRHC would begin to build a better democratic system. It would provide, too, an important journey, of the individual around themselves. For the key in an interactive, multi-media system is the last link to the end-user—how it is organised, who owns and pays for it, and on what terms. It is important to guarantee ease of access, a genuinely open network, with low-price or virtually free service. There need to be competitive pressures as different kiosk systems grow, to maximise permanent competition and diversity.

The VRHC would itself offer access by a range of information providers to consumers, since it would be both a channel and an advice centre. This would provide good clinical information, good analysis of who does what well, and on-line first-hand information from consumers, before a person agrees to a treatment. That is, vital first-hand local experiences as well as computerised databases. The VRHC would offer an opportunity to emphasise the role of pressure groups, who are already on the Net, in the public sphere. Enhanced Community Health Councils/Health Information Centres are one possible framework. This institutional innovation can be the direct and easy access to a multiplicity of providers. It will not prevent the domestic development of PC-TV interaction in the home, which will be the successor to the satellite dish as a "must have" buy. The VRHC will be the mass-market *public access point* (and training strategy) which will precede and then complement the Network computer in the front parlour. It will enter all to the real choices offered on the Internet, and emphasise the value of narrative experience to which it can connect communities, as well as assessing its difficulties. The VRHC will be an intermediary, a help with "voice", an aid with accessing, assessing, and adding to information. Of course, information is not unproblematic. The importance of guidance and support from user-groups, from librarians, perhaps from health professionals will be an issue. The VRHC will, too, encourage groups of consumers to organise *in the locality*, and it will extend the activities of user-groups marshalling international, comparative, current knowledge. Providers—which will become distribution networks themselves—will face enhanced consumer choice, insistence on elevated standards and proven content. Step-growth will be insufficient; a complete re-orientation will be required. Those with unsatisfactory access will be offered new opportunities, in a context of mutual learning. This will be a two-fold social challenge: how will the costs of empowerment be met? How will current pressures in a political marketplace for renewed local monopolies, reduced management-costs and longer-term contracts between protected providers and unaccountable purchasers be finessed?

The GP will be directly affected. The results of these initiatives, and of a VRHC, will be that both the GP and the patient would be "shopping". And with a digicash credit (as patient fundholder?) the GP knows that the patient is both shopping from him, and with him. This combination of experiences will create new levels of local consciousness about how good services are, and who is good at what. Unexpected and unacceptable variations, poor performance, will be more transparent. They will no longer be sanction-free. This will prompt rapid innovation, and re-state cultural limits. It will extend consciousness, and query "reasonableness" rationing and "affordability".

These developments enable individuals to think in global terms—where is what is best, and what is it—and to act locally. Individuals will no longer be dispersed and passive consumers. The universal access and addressing system of the WWW will enable any topic, product, service, provider, individual physician to be explored, documented, accessed, viewed on-line in a two-way discussion.

This idea for a high street multi-media, on-line community information centre is an opportunity to extend responsibility and control—rather than the detente of "partners", who are most unlikely to be of equal standing—to a large number of local communities. Effective systems of consumer representation and government regulation, requiring access and appropriate pricing (Ofhealth?), will necessarily reinforce this structure.[49]

The VRHC would have the primary task (even the primary-led task!) of assisting the public to understand the tough questions to ask of themselves and of the NHS, what to take seriously in making choices. The VRHC would make the system accountable for evidence based standards, but of standards set by patients and user-groups, in a re-definition of the evidence base of medicine. It would ask questions of evidence based distribution of services;

evidence based performance, improvement, transparency and accountability. It would be the basis of evidence based contract, incentive, and reward, and ensure organisational and management development, which is explicit and responsive, and which changes selection, socialisation and career progress in medicine. Such an approach would seek contracting for *specific* and measurable outcome, with evidence based choice.

Information and initiates: questions, quzas, and quandaries

The NHS information system remains one of initiates in command. It is a system which controls the nature of knowledge. The NHS consultative system is absorbent, and moves only a reluctant step at a time. It is a convention that skilled health professionals and managers are adept at absorbing pressure and persisting as before. Rudolf Klein, in *The Politics of the NHS*, demonstrates this throughout the history of the state system of medicine.[50] The annual reports of the Health Service Ombudsman confirm this.[51] Patient "involvement", "partnership", "listening", "choice" are each adaptable to their own purposes by any powerful group within the NHS. These consultation exercises are intended to be legitimising but they are not transforming. They are notifiable, but they are not culturally overwhelming.

The genuine template of power will be when *patients* decide how much power they have. That they have open answers to tough questions. That they control the agenda and initiate issues. That they decide what is appropriate information. That their behaviour with money impacts directly on the incomes of Chief Executives and on Doctors. That the cumulative (and even unpredictable) impact of patients' decisions changes services. This suggests that the real basis of choice and empowerment is not "partnership" on unequal terms. It is useful and useable information on clinical practice and effectiveness, evidence from patients, and organised respect for the individual (and cost-conscious) view. With both linked directly to sanction and the ability to act on that knowledge. Better information, better literature, better voice and exit, which prepares the patient for choices, advocacy and counselling. Time to consider and to take second opinions—all these are important factors in responsible citizenship and better health care. And at a time when the opportunities to benefit from new medical interventions properly carried out are unprecedented, it is of fundamental concern for the individual to get the right diagnosis promptly, then swiftly to see the clinician who they choose for the outcome they hope for and prefer. Who they judge likely to perform best within the value framework of the individual concerned and supported by what science there is. The job is to make available good science and good self. However, information—even Internet information—is not sufficient nor fully efficient. To achieve the most it is vital that the *money* does go with the patient. And that providers (together with politicians, whose hands are only ever snatched away from electrified wires) have this incentive (amongst others) to ensure that effective care is offered. This must be managed by patient-established protocols and audited by public process. It will be costly. But so is ineffective care. Public budgeting will need to gain a longer-term perspective, too.

The NHS has serious problems of how to manage innovation with social consent. Explicit rationing will further complicate this position. This is a new problem, in what Marshall Marinker recently called the "era of personal predictive medicine which will refer to the unique patient".[52] He has urged attention to a cluster of factors. Advances in IT will open up knowledge which is uncommonly shared, and ask what we mean by "knowledge". The response required has several strands. The call is for horizontal thinking across disparate disciplines; to humanise an increasingly biomechanical world; to change the current boundaries and institutions of health care. A new professional fluidity and adaptability will be required. Many existing concepts need to be seen for what they are—historical, but temporary. This is to query the very nature of public service—of how the individual relates to it, and what expectations we have not only of it but of the individual. Marshall is right. To deliver the yields of technical advance, whilst remaining sensitive to the variety of human lifestyles, we need an experimental mentality which will require quantum leaps in policy and in practice.

Whether we consider the individual as a citizen or as a consumer, these insights invite us to see that so much of the present system is unpractised, unpassionate, fundamentally lacking in intellectual and in empathetic resources and knowledge for empowering patients. The change in psychological states required is very great, if there is to be real shape and form in systems whch are appropriate to passing power to patients. For this is about the costly, challenging endeavour of everyone in the NHS giving their actions *definition* in terms of the patient's values and power. The empowerment of individual choice needs to impact on changing socialisation and assumption, and then on services. Changing "what it is like to go through this place." Changing management processes, the attitudes of staff, the speed, location and cost of services, the extent of the reach of consumer definitions of choice on clinical quality and on questions of the quality of life. These are shifts from judgments based on organisational or professional standards alone to judgments reflecting customer standards, transparently encouraged and assessed in a new kind of obviously listening audit loop.

It is clear that multi-media systems will let people discover what they need to know, what other people are able to know in other countries, and what the NHS either does not know or will not tell.

But we are asking:

We will need to ask who plans my path? What will be the likely impact of networked IT on structure, roles, professions, institutions, and present structures? What is the potential for multi-media computer networks to get us out of narrow hierarchical boxes, inherited from the world of guilds and crafts, which would take us from controlling hierarchies to open networks? These potential changes on intra-professional relations are large, as is the likely impact on professional self-interest and the political cycle in which veto organisations function.

Presently, these structural controls slow NHS development. These are problems of culture, staffing, and functioning in a political marketplace where social policy slows change. It does so in salute to ideas such as "equity", "founding values", "access" which are elusive in their meaning, application, and outcome. Here, we confront the necessity to re-define roles, language, expectations. Take roles. A key change will be in primary care. What do we mean by "the GP" and "the patient"? The cultural answers are less obvious than they were. Clearly, each may be better informed, in order to be better informing. For the "GP", information and work (and hence training?) will be much more community-based. There are many pressures to prompt us to examine the development of a generic health-worker in an advisory role. One possibility is the "GP" as geographer, as problem-solver, as "pilot" chosen by the individual as the person on which they wish to rely for guidance. This is the healthworker helping people to visualise potential pathways as choices. This idea is that the GP will become an outreach networker in multi-media. The GP's role will be, as agent, to try to move up the value-chain, working with clients and alongside them in making choices through the net. They will, together, work the electronic marketplace. And the GP will have to prove that they know how, and get good results. The GP is at present both a proxy agent (for the patient, requiring hospital services), a middle manager and a distributor–provider, on behalf of its client, the government. The role of the GP is to develop as a true, high-quality intermediary. This would greatly affect traditional relationships and replace many tasks currently performed by GPs alone. It would shift many clinical tasks. It would possibly give greater value to non-clinical knowledge, with important re-definitions of professional activity. To achieve this within the professions a new consensus of what can be handed on needs to be explicitly addressed.

The GP has controlled costs, rationed services, acted as first point of call, functioned as link or mediator between producer and consumer. GPs have been paid transaction fees for this proxy and advisory role, and have undertaken the key role of initial diagnosis and advice in a relationship of trust, advocacy and solidarity. But as information becomes widely available, these roles will need to develop further. So, too, will the entire practice team, to help patients find their own paths. Particularly so, as chronic care predominates, and as patients need to be trained and supported to use new technologies. Carers, increasingly important, will be closely linked by IT. These changes offer a mutual learning experience with the individual as their own case-manager. They stress again the importance of the information agent, the advocate in guidance on individual autonomy and choice. This idea offers a new notion of balance between information, agent, and the individual patient/service user.

Iona Heath, in *The Mystery of General Practice*, has said that the GP is at the interface between illness and disease where the vast undifferentiated mass of human distress meets the theoretical structures of scientific medicine and social science. Here, we still know too little about understanding and controlling the experience of illness. It is Heath's view that it is the GP's chief job to help the patient understand, and to cope with this. This is the "biographic role" proposed by Marshall Marinker.[53] Here, there is still too much focus on science, on "objective" facts. The medical model captures us in damaging cultural perspectives. These exclude the patient's special knowledge and values. These exclude the potential for self-responsibility, self-knowledge, self-care, coping with our principal burden of chronic disease in the community, and of long-term mental health care.

It seems likely that multi-media will increase the primacy of primary care in a multi-tiered delivery system in which computers fully integrate care. The balkanisation and fragmentation of medicine by specialty will also be reintegrated. It will also offer a new vehicle for negotiation with the community, as medicine re-emphasises its responsibilities to quality.

However, it is not self-evident that the education and training, and the recent re-focusing of interest by GPs, makes them necessarily the best agent for the patient. There is an issue of how alternative intermediaries might be developed. Here, some user groups offer themselves for this role. The GP, as an intermediate institution, remains un-transparent and un-accountable. We need, too, a vocabulary for the measurement of performance, service and quality. The paradox is that the GP is the one who the public trusts as a source of information, yet its availability might undermine professional trust. In addition, information might prompt exit, but there is as yet no satisfactory entrance elsewhere. The power of incumbency, the costs of market entrance, the social peer group pressures which constrain competition, have, too, been increased by the multi-fund concept.

One of the great social challenges is, of course, that improvements in acute care enable more people to survive into older age characterised by chronic conditions. Medicine generates its own excruciating paradoxes and frustrations. Many arise from its greatest successes. Success in one field has transferred the problem elsewhere. Thus, the successes of emergency medicine and acute care have produced the challenge of long-term care. Thus, intractable, progressive, degenerative problems, chronic care problems (which, of course, can have acute episodes). Hospital medicine can deal with acute episodes without halting the progression of the disease. Survival has been achieved at the price of the need to live with difficult to manage conditions. For many this implies a sicker life with a poor quality of life. Now, as Edward Tenner has emphasised in an exceptional analysis, the instruments and concepts of the late 20th century have shifted our attention to the cumulative impact of those things which can be imperceptibly gradual, but which do not go away. We can detect the early stages of long-duration problems: "We can measure substances in concentrations, once too minute to detect. We can capture patterns once inaccessible or hopelessly blurred. We can not only measure present conditions but extrapolate future ones. All these abilities raise gradual processes to a new level of concern. They make them as real, and as catastrophic in their implications, as high-impact events."[54]

We usually come late to the chronic. These conditions require special and expensive skills which are in short supply. They can be helped by new technology, but with a fundamental ambivalence: for this requires more training, both of doctor and patient, not less; more professional commitment, not less; more patient understanding and engagement, not less; greater expenditure, to give back-up. It is a mixed message. It is possible to be healthier than ever, yet more anxious. Health can indeed be a form of paranoia. Health indicators tell a positive story, the individual's mind a negative tale. Peace of mind is nudged by escalating costs, by a new focus on symptoms and amplified dangers, greater cultural understanding and understanding of iatrogenic effects, the multiplication of disabling dependency, and by the reduction of the leeway that people are wont to concede to a suffering individual, as Ivan Illich pointed out. In Aaron Wildavsky's phrase, we are "doing better but feeling worse."[55]

Chronic illnesses set us apart from one another. Anselm L. Strauss, the medical sociologist, has clarified the characteristics on which policy attention needs to focus. Chronic illnesses are socially divisive; they are a major strain on the suffering individual, on families, and on resources. They are long-term by their nature; uncertain in prognosis; demand relatively more symptomatic relief, which can be costly; they are multiple diseases, in which one systems breakdown can damage others; they are socially disruptive for patients and their carers and communities; they call for a variety of social and community as well as medical services, and they are expensive.[56] Here, multi-media technology has another special and liberating contribution to make—in maintaining contact with patients in their homes, in monitoring those most at risk, in enabling electronic aids to be used for home care. Survivors of catastrophic injury, or those living with congenital conditions or the results of acute interventions, can benefit from new ways of accessing their humanity. Multi-media computers and peripherals enable users to take part in a host of activities, to scan, read, recognise speech, and even synthesise their own speech.

The individual patient will increasingly become a key part of the home-performance team. This is a necessary consequence of chronic care, and of the need for vigilance in home care in which the patient is more responsibly involved. Interactive home computer links will offer guidance on how to give drugs, what to do if a child has a seizure, how to watch for side-effects, including machine signals when a patient is allergic to a drug. They will give individuals personal health checks, provide guidance from a home database, prime doctors on which kinds of patients do well on which therapies. They will, too, give guidance to health workers on what might be a problem for a particular patient, based on digitised records which extract more from patient records on what to do, what a symptom might mean. One of the greatest challenges of chronic care is home care, which can become a full-time task, imposing big burdens on carers and on costs. Tenner points out that much of the task of health care in the future may not be magic breakthroughs but maintenance, holding on to what we have gained: "As we advance, we look back, and watch the shadows over our shoulders reforming in new ways. We will move ahead but must always look back just because reality is indeed gaining on us."[57]

The more advanced medicine and surgery becomes, the more demanding it is in requiring training, vigilance, skilled craftsmanship and dexterity. Avoiding serious error requires greater attention on the part of physicians, surgeons, nurses, technicians—and patients. And, increasingly, of computer programmers and software developers, since machinery controlled by software can malfunction in control of key processes. Those tests which are made automatic and which are digitised may prompt too great a reliance on what the machine "says". Here, noticing a problem, querying a result, having a hunch, following intuition, valuing "art" can be vital. Here practice can make nearer to perfect, and can help an individual assess whether results look right—to avoid false positive and unreliable results. This, again, is a twin burden—new technological competence and old style alertness; the patient helped, the patient challenged.

The interaction between patients on networks will query another given. This concerns the emphasis on curative medicine and its over-stated powers. This emphasis is deeply harmful since it helps create expectations of an un-doable job. That is, that there is an objective cure for all diseases and for all patients. This shuts out our "inside", or psycho–social reality. The emphasis on disease and on scientific objectivity denies the "knowledge", the soft-facts about self, about quality of life, about preferred outcomes. This especially interferes with successful chronic management. Mystery has to be opened up, to help doctors as much as to help patients. There is a need for doctors to explain themselves, to define practice and priorities, to debate with patients the limitations as well as the possibilities of medicine, and to make choices supportable and explicit. Nor are all our health decisions about life or death issues; many are life-style choices. This requires the confession and sharing of uncertainty, and the recognition that death is not optional. Nor are doctors necessarily to blame. We need, instead, to focus on two things: the real sources of sickness, and the different contributions that medicine and the patient can make. Robert Evans, as we know, speaks of disease as an *expression*. What we now know, but do not act upon, needs more thoughtful attention, as Evans demonstrates.

Crucially, the job is to narrow the performance range of processes, to optimise care, as innovative purchasers of care like Dr Harry Burns in Glasgow has emphasised.[58] Yet in asking which is the right procedure, values are routinely under-valued. And this is a determinant of outcome which is not being measured. Doctors need this comparative data too, to inform themselves about their performance by comparison with others. How are they doing? How good am I? How could I get better? Where am I on the distribution curve? The average is not necessarily virtuous. In assessing the problems of risk, benefit, distribution, averages, and probability, patients and doctors will need training if they are to be able to answer whether it will help to know more and can you benefit. Health authorities buy care for "populations" and rely on distribution curves. Yet the individual patient shies from this epic to the intimate, and wants a specific number. This is not on offer. Instead, best probabilistic models give general ranges. How sure then is it worth being about a diagnosis—is it worth the cost-pay-off? How to use networked data—and the shared assumptions of exploring these together—to explore how a patient evaluates risk, and the potentially hazardous clinical environment? Samuel Brittan has reminded us of the difference between risk and uncertainty. Risks are calculable and insurable; uncertainty occurs when you do not know what the risks are and cannot estimate the likelihood of any particular outcome. However, in most situations you can obtain some vague idea of magnitudes. There is a spectrum between pure risk and utter uncertainty.

In many situations, patients can come to judgments which they make about what they are prepared to accept.[59]

The Changing Provider: Value-chains, visionaries, and virtual systems

The starting point of transformation is the business model. That is, the high-level abstraction of what the business is, how it can respond to and create markets, what the business is and could be, what value-added will the users and customers want? There is a transformation in management thinking required, which is to shift from deductive to inductive thinking, to find the solution and apply it to a problem.

Relatively structured business processes will be re-examined, since knowledge work will be based on accessing skills wherever they are located. Computing links between enterprises are beginning to blur traditional boundaries between organisations. Hospitals increasingly use digital transfers, and then teleconference with consultants when expert diagnosis is required. The new network links are enabling new kinds of business relationships among organisations. Networks are extending the geographic range and market penetration of organisations, transforming the nature of business, interactions, and, necessarily, business strategy.

This accelerating shift will give the competitive edge to knowledge-based activity and will give doctors greater leverage in an expert market. The firm as we know it is breaking up. Instead, effective individuals, working in high-performance team structures, are becoming integrated organisational affinity groups. In the wider economy, this is changing the way products and services are created, marketed, and distributed. In health systems, clinical directorates of business units will be networked, and will view themselves as a unit within a modular and flexible organisation. As they respond to telemedicine opportunities and networked multi-media contact they will develop entrepreneurially.

A consumer-enterprise culture will enable business operations to be transformed, and new leaders to come forward. Specialists will strengthen themselves against generalists; NHS managers will revert to facilitation roles; aside from specialists, pay differentials will narrow. Management—probably by doctors—will guide flexible teams and networks. The people who will come out top in the new provider organisations will be the key creators or analysts who "link" their own brains with multi-media technology, to develop new medical services, new products, new link-ups. These will be doctors who can combine medical knowledge with managerial and complex networking ability, and who have the personal capacity to shift their cultural references. The old model of leadership focused on a single individual will be replaced by a networked, virtual leadership of team skills, with challenged, empowered, excited, appropriately rewarded people. Vision will be transmitted upwards from the front-line, too, with a good chance of being implemented in Zuboff's "informated" organisation. The key power of personal multi-media is its role in creating high-performance, networked linked teams, which cut across traditional organisational boundaries. This is the concept of "the platform approach", the organisational and management concept which uses networks to bring all relevant skills together. In this "value chain" people and enterprises reach out through technology to their customers, suppliers, affinity groups, and even competitors.

Exchanges between public organisations are becoming digital. And therefore open to analysis in new ways. Systems themselves are extending outside organisations to customers, suppliers, partners, competitors—providing timely information, reducing costs, increasing transaction speeds, recording and analyzing everything. Work and action is ceasing to be linear; the premium is on flexibility, innovation, entrepreneurship, and the ability to form flexible partnerships. Using telepresence, people connect on networks verbally, facially, with body language, with paperwork, pictures, sounds, all the signalling-equipment for electronic network to build leadership. Selection, socialisation, training and lifelong learning are fundamental now, in practice as well as in theory. High performance follows integrated, networked, open, and client-service networking. Low or unassessed performance; unintegrated services; host-based and proprietary monopoly provision will go into the margins. As will management by hierarchy, command and control.

The distant visualisation of data and images, with real-time animation and virtual-reality systems, will globalise a proportion of diagnosis and treatment. This area of tactile sensing is, however, in its infancy. Long-distance surgery is presently hampered in its development by patient anxiety, and by concerns about costs and security. The key will remain a relationship of solidarity with a hands-on adviser. The technical achievement presently, too, runs ahead of an economically viable mainstream. Fundamental changes are beginning to occur. Remote delivery for patient records, radiology, dermatology, pathology and continuing medical education are opening the doors, if slowly. The medium-term prospect must be, however, that there will be great changes in relationships between and within health care organisations. One consequence may be that hierarchical business models will break down into "informated" teams—involved teams, who want to do the job well, and want to communicate with their customers.[60] Another consequence may be that there will be a further loosening of the individual's commitment to "place", already a distinctive 20th century phenomenon.

As computing, communications, content, and customer converge, databases will transform many specialist roles. As service users communicate directly through e-mail, desk-top multi-media, user bulletin-board groups, and other interactive multi-media, inherited organisational architectures will fail. The information function and thus core management will be re-aligned with the customer's wishes. Here, work and learning will become integrated. As Tapscott says, "There is a new hierarchy of promise—the effective individual, the high-performance team, the integrated organisation, the extended enterprise—all cascading upward to create a new model for the creation of wealth: the internet-worked business".[61] For we are on the threshold of a virtual and digital real-time world in which producers will be expected to create specific services to meet the wishes of individual customers.

There will be new virtual services, new customer-focused structures, new roles for employees motivated to deliver this new framework. In the emergency environment, BT's CamNet project enables pictures of an accident victim to be sent to emergency doctors from a headset worn by a paramedic. The training opportunities for junior doctors are valuable. Ambulance and A&E staffs, surgeons and generic health workers will conduct consultations with distant specialists. Kent Ambulance NHS Trust is piloting a remote patient monitoring system. We can expect that ambulances will use CD ROM databases to pre-select the most appropriate centre to which to take an emergency case; each will have the patient's Health-Record Digicard, and swipe it through a reader to access all records held on a patient's health history. For an emergency case, this will be especially important—it will show history, allergic reactions, advance directives, pre-existing conditions, next of kin, and access GP guidance. New network linkages can standardise practice, improve adherence to standards, enhance performance, reduce unnecessary surgery and dangerous drug regimes, improve cost controls. The challenge is to achieve linkages without stunting the innovation that derives from competition and the expression of flair. Technological changes suggest there will be constantly changing alliances within and between provider units, as the sharing of information reveals alternative possibilities. We need the benefits of successful integration, without fossilising the present in a political marketplace. We need to halt unnecessary care and its costs, and access the under-used. We need to manage the irrational into the margin, and give incentives to the best leadership in clinical disciplines. We need a cost-effective system, not a structure of isolated republics. We need what multi-media internet-working may offer: managed care led by the most effective individual practitioners, fronting teams that integrate skills both local and distant, who contribute their knowledge and new learning to others throughout the growing information infrastructure.

This patient–enterprise architecture will need to transform business operations and the health service's information strategy around these perspectives. For walls within and around organisations are coming down, as organisations network in partnerships, uniting their core competencies and talents with the complementary competencies of others. These alliances will be impermanent, and reshaped as markets and demands alter. Information systems will be the enabler of these new business relationships. This is an issue concerning capital resources. Electronic systems for meeting customer's wishes are reaching outside the core organisation, to work on their behalf with others, including competitors. The method is the digital network. This model achieves partnerships without changes in stockholding, shareholding, ownership, capital investment. It will make more economic sense to network than to buy other people's assets. The potential is for improved medical decision-making, greater productivity, and enhanced cost-effectiveness. The ambition will be best-quality services, at lowest costs, in locations which allow easy access to patients—supported by on-line access to the best services anywhere in the world. A hospital's radiology network, for example, may consist of senior doctors at several medical centres, who "meet" patients through the World Wide Web. As Tapscott points out, Michael Porter's value chain transforms into a value network, to generate new symbiotic value in flexible, entrepreneurial relationships.[62]

The place of work, for some medical interventions, will be the system, not the place. Technologies integrated across an organisation and extended outside connect individuals who can function in new ways as a team: specialist skills, GPs, customers at home, carers, community support teams will all be linked electronically. Health care systems may parallel the system established by THISCO (The Hotel Industry Switch Company) in the USA, which, since 1989, has linked every major hotel chain to travel agents and airlines terminals. Initially, THISCO linked 340 000 airline terminals and 24 000 hotel properties, with direct on-line networking. Technology is forcing hotel chains to compete where they didn't have to in the same ways before. Virtual shopping, competitive services, comments on the Net by other guests, every detail checkable—beds, staff, privacy, environment, noise levels, no smoking policies, parking, transportation, privacy and ambience, on-line discussions, all of which established relationships or deny them. All of which creates quality control data in an electronic marketplace.[63] The NHS equivalent would include virtual presentation of mixed wards, and of private facilities. Markets are becoming electronic as products become digital and networked.

Tapscott says: 'What matters in every case is that the new technologies can transform not only business processes but also the way products and services are created and marketed, the structure and goals of the enterprise, the dynamics of competition, and the actual nature of the enterprise."[64] Survival for an organisation will be about value-added opportunities. This will include being orientated so that improved customer service is everyone's daily test—with each employee understanding its significance.

IT is changing internal structures to get the job done. Intranet systems—internal networks based on Internet standards—will also take advantage of the open protocols, standards, and the familiar Web browser software of the public Internet to provide employees, customers and suppliers with easy access to corporate information and processes, to be more open and responsive to patients. This development will offer the NHS a special benefit: it will consolidate the patchwork of incompatible computer systems, software, and databases which characterise NHS computing investment. To realise networked benefits providers will need to develop the capability to integrate or buy integrated systems that will connect users to others within the enterprise, that will connect all users to vital data and information, that will connect everyone to potential customers, to suppliers, and to networked partners.

The initial key is client/server computing. The Intranet is the internal black box which will seek to integrate the enterprise, on the desktop. The provider must get several things right—components, system platforms, connectivity software and client/services. *Attitude* is above all important; and it is attitude which is the biggest problem throughout the NHS. These shifts and investments in power-hungry 64-bit high performance computing are a requirement in business applications such as multi-media, visualisation, simulation and modelling which are essential to medicine and to interactive video servers. This will be truly competitive differentiation—even if the political market seeks to restrict its operation. Scalable systems will need to be there, to enable human-scale services which people want to access, and which they can do so on their own terms and in terms of their own values. The key is that many activities, like those of so-called knowledge workers, are not as dependent on time and place and will be decoupled from geography much sooner. The advantages are in off-line processing, time-shifting, and access to the very best. The NHS provider will have to move up the power curve, which will be increasingly visible to the ordinary consumer adept at the Net. These systems will be wanted by doctors who want to network, providers who want to offer new networked skills, and to achieve competitive advantage, and management controls in finance.

The NHS does not serve the end consumer. It serves the customers of its customers. In a networked world it will need to search out the end user, as well as helping the existing proxy agent to help their customers. The networked NHS provider will be thus a creative influence in the digital economy. It will be equipped to respond when distant customers search out its own services. The capability of customers will change and improve; the job of the provider is to capture that capability, for mutual ends.

The key is to operate competitive capability, not functions alone. User choice and information will have to be fully aligned. If you don't do it, new players, new partnerships, new niche players, new hybrid organisations, new networks will seek to do so instead. It will be the core network and the computing infrastructure which will be key to seamless, consistent services which people want to pay for. Personnel Directors must be big cats in this jungle, since it is attitudes and ways of working which must change most—what the management literature calls "the legacy cultures". Personnel must cease to be a functional orientation, and become a customer orientation, with an external not an internal view. The world of one size fits nobody—of undifferentiated mass access—will no longer serve. It is not sufficient to get better without changing. NHS Trusts will only be secure within their borders if they extend them globally. Multi-media technology will change diagnosis, and its location; delivery, and its teams; management structures, and its purposes; relationships between doctors, managers, and patients. Networks will empower both patients and professionals, and shift the rules of performance, incentive, contract, and financial structures in the political marketplace. This will not necessarily imply a decrease in complexity. Indeed, it may well result in the opposite if a provider seeks to do business across geographic boundaries, and to liberate its specialist teams to link with others to provide services globally.

Mark Twain's obituary? The end of the era of the hospital

Like Twain's reported demise, the end of the hospital has often been prematurely reported. But the new digital quietus may ensure we see the end of the era of the hospital as the locus of health care delivery. Instead, we will see a competitive managed-care environment and integrated, networked delivery systems often provided outside the walls of the hospital. The temptation to own buildings or to employ doctors on long contracts will be resistible. Development will be achieved electronically, without costly asset-based integration.

The Hospital will give way to a system that will cater to the wishes of its customers by offering a variety of services, networked through a variety of vendors in an integrated delivery plan. Hospitals are technologically obsolete. As networked systems change the role of the consumer they will—in a political marketplace where health is about votes—become politically obsolete too. A successful virtual health system will need clients, capital, committed and skilled staff, information technology, and market power.

It will be more difficult to be a doctor, it will be harder to manage market share, utilisation, risk-sharing, cost and re-imbursement. It will be more challenging to be a potential patient. It will be interesting to be a politician. The basic indicators will be measured, published, compared: choice, cost, access, quality, outcome, patient satisfaction. Leverage for the provider will be rooted in multi-disciplinary skills, as the basis of organisational effectiveness. Small teams will be responsible for competitive positioning. The model will be integrated networks and delivery systems. A modern hospital has many networked systems. There are personal multi-media devices for diagnostic and 3-D visualisation, to improve the effectiveness of individual health workers. There are new multi-media workstations. There are collaborative computing environments for teams using interactive clinical information systems, including links with carers and community-based care teams. The future is for an integrated health care delivery system, which extends across a major hospital or series of hospitals, or across an entire health purchasing area where value-driven action must replace cost-based buying decisions. Providers will need to become virtual health care systems. This will bring together all records, all teams, all healthworkers, linked by an integrated patient-based record to enhance seamless care. This will digitalise test results, lab. reports, operating room information, medication profiles, radiology reports, discharge data, personal information, costing, and external standards. Community and regional networks will link the GP to the available alternative referral centres, and the local hospital to the major sites, teaching hospitals, specialist centres—sharing information in collaborative working also. They will also link with local outpatient and inpatient systems and social services. There will be national linkages, connections to national effectiveness and research databases, and other central data. The ambition of seamless care will be assisted by technological links which will help patients move through the system cost-effectively and kindly. Technology is an important part of the solution to the critical medical manpower shortage, linking things, calling in opinion from distance. Networks may also encourage early screening and intervention, and integrate the patient into the team on a life-long basis. For the successful provider will have direct or strategic partnerships with long-term care provision, nursing homes, home-care support, and family practice, all internetworked. Capitation provision within agreed care-plan budgets and internetworked services may combine to change structures profoundly.[65]

We need, too, to use new media to measure patient satisfaction, to measure every transaction in terms of the customer's expectations and satisfaction, which will change the balance between what people want and what is wanted by the central authorities. We need clear measures of service quality, from the customer's perspective. This means helping the patient to know the key questions to ask us. This information should be collected and distributed in the local community, and kept current on the Internet. This is the key process in achieving and in re-defining success for good teams, which always include the customers. It would be a good beginning to start by measuring the 10 events which most disappoint and frustrate customers, with each weighted from a customer perspective on a 10-point scale. Here, integrated and networked new technology can achieve improvements, by scanning five areas: scanning and monitoring physical systems and the environment; monitoring transactions in information and financial systems; monitoring direct-contact systems which directly support customers; monitoring what professionals do; gathering and publishing what users tell of their experiences. This is to situate technology around quality goals. It is also to use comparison reports to improve services, and to spot problems before there is a failure from the perspective of the customer. This requires a management view of continuous learning and action, using information technology in continuous accounting. None of this will work if those at the "bottom" are viewed as "erks". For everyone has to understand information technology and customer service, what the information is, why, and how it is used. Everyone has to become a leader, with decisions placed in the hands of people all the way down the organisation. A necessary sequence of digital architecture is to empower employees with multiple skills, with data, with incentive, and with both authority and an understanding of where what they do fits into the broader processes. A fundamental is to discover/teach what "an improvement" would be, as a specific change, as Leigh Richardson has stressed.

Doctors and medical colleagues are in the front line, not least in enhancing the only sustainable advantage, which is organisational consciousness and learning to achieve proven quality outputs determined in advance. Technology is re-defining roles. Here, the job is to empower the front-line to make more decisions and respond successfully to customer wishes and problems. The job is to build the retailing model of concern and responsiveness into public services. The job is to create a consumer-led NHS, by providing services from the consumer's point of view. Smart-cards will be very significant. These raise major concerns of privacy, security, status of personal information and of how it might be used. These also raise potential opportunities for informing consumers, and empowering them to exert leverage. These are questions of personal control and "smart privacy", which can be creative and which will be important themes in public policy debates. As Perri 6 and Ivan Briscoe have said: "Smart-cards will be the first and most tangible and the most visible focus for these debates."[66] Smartcards will change information politics, and will be the citizen's portable key to the information economy and to many basic services. Health care promises to be one of the most important and beneficial fields for their use, with many benefits in principle offered to empower the user. It suggests beneficial and fruitful collaborative possibilities between technology and user wants. In health care, the Exmouth Health Care Card has had a positive trial, and there are health, social and health insurance cards being issued or trialled in France, Germany, Spain, Canada, Australia and New Zealand.[67] The prospect is of prompt European-wide convergence in standards and usage. Smart cards will integrate the customer into the management and delivery of services. At last, there will be an effective patient information director who integrates the range of fragmented patient response services—literature, appointments, clinic times, parking arrangements, Patients Charter, outcomes data. The patient is an essential part of the solution—holding smart card patient-held records. These can hold all patient records, and can be linked to digicash billing systems. They will be credit, debit and access cards, the entry to value networks. They will co-exist and seem normal, alongside smart clothes (holding manufacturing and sales memory), smart houses (for environmental control), smart roads (for monitoring, mapping, safety, and pricing), smart cars (integrating driving performance and operation), and smart electronics (interactive, personal multi-media). Technology will rapidly eliminate "host-based" systems, which look inwards. The future is customer-based systems, which look outwards so that in an important empowered sense the customers run the business. It is necessary to do more than create new services.

The job is to transform the entire organisation, its nature and culture, its approach and its quality. In business terms, as Paul Hodgkin has said, "the creative place consists of being off balance, just ahead of the wave, projecting into the future".[68] In patient terms, as John Simmonds has said, the creative place to be is at the letter-box and where patient stories are being told. It is essential that as professionals claim their special authority in a system of interactive media, patient expertise and knowledge is recognised, with institutions in place to empower them to set the context for professional work.

The Beginning, at The End: Austen's dizzy heroine

There are other questions to examine. These mirror stubborn and problematic conflicts of interest. For example as we build data, who owns the information? Who collects, organises and censors it? There is already an issue of who owns the patient records. How to resolve issues of access, price, charging, copyright, regulation, investment and return? Will there be a charge for putting information into networks and for taking it out? When I share information am I impoverished by it or enriched by it? Will research centres be charged, or charge? We revert constantly to questions of power, hierarchy, and control. What will the professionals and politicians allow us to know and openly debate—both in the presentation of information, and in the values and structures of the ideas behind it? What is to be included, excluded, or denied? What will we refuse, as citizens and as consumers to allow "them" to deny "us"? How will we ensure that safety comes from multiple inputs—from professionals and from the individual. Will this be resolved, expressed in terms of what the system will allow in, or by a de-centralised, democratic structure? Will politicians, social policies, Royal Colleges, institutions and stakeholders assist or restrict the process of change? How will they hinder/prompt information technology? How will new professional roles emerge? As each step is taken government, as regulator, will have to make the ethical and operational rules and respond to social pressures to make new ones.

There will be a challenge, and possibly a crisis, of leadership in our organisations. Every organisation will have to be more open to leadership for transformation, and not turn their back on change. Such shifts of a paradigm nature involve dislocation, conflict, confusion, and uncertainty, such that the established leaders are the last to be won over, if at all. The key will be create trust, but based on allowing patient views, ideas, and experiences into the structure in ways that are persuasive and compelling, and in ways which empower those who want to hear. This will be very difficult indeed as technology enhances insecurity. Yet professionals, as the ultimate knowledge workers and as one important kind of intellectual asset, need not lose their status. This will, however, will have to be supported by proven performance to international standards which are set by customers, and by the openness to listening and to empowering the individual. The key asset is not fixed capital—which can be rented, and managed—but knowledge. This, as I have argued, has many homes. The measurement and management of both fixed, networked, and patient-held assets will need to change, guided by the imperative of openness and improvement. Capital will be a function of knowledge; knowledge will come from users as much as from professionals; knowledge will open and published. The ability to retain and enhance the diverse knowledge capability of the open, networked system will provide security and the necessary base for innovation and creativity. If not, current or future competitors will overwhelm those who believe it is sufficient to improve on an unchanged structure. If all share the same technology, if all services can be copied, who crosses the line first?

We could recall Langdon Winner. And pay regard to what Neil Belton recently said, that "English culture is full of antiquated barricades, tollgates at crossing points between forms of imagination that should be free and open."[69] Technology has unsettling power, too, in its ability to disrupt our image of our own past and of the nearby future. In its capacity to stir new thoughts, new anxieties, fear and promise, in ways which overleap the traditional divide between science and culture.[70] The point, however, is that we *can* invent a different answer which becomes the orientation of the entire system. We can benefit from multimedia innovation provided we have a philosophy of technology rooted in a philosophy of open being, which is intimate with a philosophy of choice and of liberty. It is a considerable psychological shift. It is necessary, too, to recognise that it is political will, not patient incapacity, which restrains us, which prevents empowerment from being a continent and not merely a coastline. We need to choose our structures, techniques, and efficiencies from a different point of view.

It is easy to be uneasy. It is easy to doubt the potentials for change. Costs, clearly, will be considerable. Yet the price of not changing is not to be dismissed, even when costs are budgeted in the insular NHS style of year in year only. Empowerment of the individual is necessary if trumping aces are to be played to improve health care, and to influence its determinants. In terms of cultural transformation this will depend upon and reinforce an optimistic view of human character and potential. It will disseminate the special transforming powers of choice in society. It will endorse the self-management of chronic care, and re-focus support for those experiencing mental illness.[71] Empowerment is essential, too, if the patient is successfully to use new and complex medical technology at home. For new health technologies will not necessarily make life less complicated; they require trained understanding. Much more care will become the responsibility of the user, routinely video-conferencing, linked by computers for electronic health-checks and supportive advice. This is the essential orientation and focus of modern health care where long term care is getting longer, and is chiefly chronic care in the community. Health care need not be experienced as hierarchy and control, but as active coping in ones own terms. This is the essential focus for a consumer-led service in each aspect of health care. This is what the NHS needs to stretch to deliver. To recognise and be orientated around patients as the source of special and unique knowledge in a democracy, rather than around the claims of the special role that "expert" knowledge ought to play. Here, much of the most important evidence must come *from* patients and users *to* professionals. This is to call for change management in terms of the power of the patients' experience. For new ways of listening and seeing, to turn information into both internal and external knowledge; to turn knowledge into selection by patients; with devices for leverage to empower, to ensure that knowledge truly *is* power. Based on knowledge of user experiences, which is the link and context for different kinds of expertise, and the necessary protection for deep cultural diversity.

W. E. Gladstone wrote: "It is better to write one word upon the rock than a thousand on the water or the sand." And, as Darwin said in the closing words of *The Origin of Species*, "from so simple a beginning, endless forms most beautiful and most wonderful have been, and are being evolved."[72] We are on the threshold of a huge cultural shift, in which there could be a much more aware (if not necessarily a much more "sophisticated") patient. One in which there can be a different configuration of socialisation and of skills, disciplines and services. One in which the values of both professionals and patients can be effectively engaged with a new agenda as we explore the major public policy issue of discovering what really goes on, of how to be open to listening to discover it, and of how to renovate health care, self-management, and voluntary association.

These arguments are all about what Joyce in *Ulysses* calls "those big words . . . which make us so unhappy".[7] That is, belief and faith, power, control, freedom, choice, responsibility, community, leadership, and outcome. And, most notably in a world of huge technological shifts, culture and cultural policy. Yet each needs to be understood, and properly situated, in considering the future of healthcare. And a cultural policy is a requirement if the ends of any public policy are to be achieved. For, in the NHS context, culture should not merely be invoked in recognition of difficulty. Instead, it is central to the changes required in a democracy. Indeed, as Perri 6 has pointed out: "Creating and sustaining the cultural resources necessary to make privately based economic dynamism and social viability possible is the central task for a society. In other words the most important task of government is to make it possible for a society to organise itself."[74]

Fundamental to how we can successfully organise healthcare in the modern context is the ability of the user of health services to build their own understandings in a system where many roles must change. That is, their capacity to apply information, facts, concepts, skills, and knowledge in new and appropriate situations. Here, I have argued, we need much more thought about the relationship between information and knowledge, so that service users can "hear" the information in ways in which they can use it, learn with it and from it. For, in medicine, "knowledge" relates critically to "outcome". It is this, and not "information" (or activity), which is the product.

To make such progress, it is necessary to actively support the user to ask the NHS provider very difficult questions which it has preferred to overlook. And to work with answers that clients determine they can live with. The necessity is to transfer expertise to clients, so that they can build their capacity to *select*, to learn, to share questions, to discuss ideas and knowledge, to contribute to outcomes. To borrow from Joyce: "It must be a movement then, an actuality of the possible as possible."[75] And this as an alternative to the bureaucratic frame of mind, to what he calls "the pluterperfect imperturbability of the Department of Agriculture." This is to identify a very large project. It is to start again from first principles. This offers not an either/or antithesis, but a both/and philosophy, for each of us in our plurality of identities. In fact, whether unhappy with big words or not, technology has changed the situation in ways which Stephen Dedalus, Buck Mulligan, Mr Deasy, Cissy Caffree, Mrs Breen, Father Conmee, Mr Bloom et al would find deeply astonishing, whether in Dublin or anywhere and in all future worlds. It seems very likely that a UK "market" of 57 million people will attract investment by Microsoft, Toshiba, Toyota and others in software resources which offer guidance on disease, treatments, risks, benefits, narrative opinion, probability, and outcome together with information on who does what well. Who will justify the redemptive trust required to help people use such resources?

At the same time, there is the political requirement for the system to be much more accountable. This will be met by interactive multimedia. Healthcare will be scrutinised in terms of the trinity of management accountability, public accountability, and personal accountability. Faced with these three articulate Foxes, Brer Rabbit (born and bred in the briar patch of aggregate data) will now need to run a different and more specific race. The aggregate and individual will be distinguished and transparently accountable. For this is the distinction between giving an account and being held to account, both by the local community (for "strategy") and by the individual user (for what works). The services, too, will recruit from fundamental behavioural skills as well as medical and managerial abilities.

The most persuasive impact of new technologies is, of course, where it flows with those cultural shifts which already form a waterfall. These are the torrents of greater international competition and transparency, and of greater self-reliance. Towards choice and liberty and away from dependence on professionals, away from myth, mystique and mystery. It is these global changes which form the context within which effective leadership is required, and where the expression of strength of purpose is essential. It is this which will form the Future, Joyce's "Sister of the Past".

This is to shift from a view of the patient as someone who cuts a poor figure in a doctor's journal—someone like the Bertram girls in *Mansfield Park*, unequal in "rank, fortune, rights and expectations." It is to displace someone like the disregarded Fanny, who, though "often mortified by their treatment of her, [she] thought too lowly of her own claims to feel injured by it". This is to adjust the emphasis from someone much like Austen's dizzy heroine, the "almost pretty" Catherine Morland of *Northanger Abbey*, who, though hastening to perfect felicity, "never could learn anything before she was taught, and sometimes not even then, for she was often inattentive, and occasionally stupid."[76] Instead, we license Jane Austen's preference for reconciliation in narrative, but on post-modernist terms in the age of hyper-text and of the story of patient power. For we do not live in a Regency parkland, nor in a quiet Hampshire village vicarage of little pieces of ivory. Instead, in the global and conspicuously transparent world of changing health care, being digital is to listen best, not to know best. It is to discover avenues for patients to speak about their experiences, to the service, to one another, and to themselves. It is to devise devices which empower them. It is for the NHS to accept Elizabeth Bennett's remark, while dancing with Mr Darcy at Netherfield Ball, that "I must not decide upon my own performance." It is, too, to admit the difficulty identified by Yeats, of the courage a man may show in "entering the abyss of himself." The NHS might then say: "Praise us as we are tasted, allow us as we prove; our heads shall go bare 'til merit crown us."[77]

Acknowledgements: I am indebted for a number of discussions on these issues shared with Professor Marshall Marinker, and with John Simmonds. I am also grateful to Professor AJ Cullyer, Dr Paul Hodgkin, Adam Darkins, Dr David G Green, Rick Nye, Perri 6, Ray Rowden, and Leigh Richardson, for our conversations on the topics reviewed here.

1 I am also especially beholden for my understanding of these issues to John Simmonds (formerly Chairman of Brighton Health Authority) for our discussions as friends and colleagues over many years. Also, to Dr David Green (Director of the Institute of Economic Affairs Health & Welfare Unit). The Flaubert reference is from Gustave Flaubert, *The Dictionary of Received Ideas*, trans Geoffrey Wall, London, Syrens, Penguin, 1994; The Asian references are from Paul Theroux, *The Great Railway Bazaar*, London, Hamish Hamilton, 1975; Penguin edition, 1977, p 175, p 188. On "la technique", see Jacques

Ellul, *The Technological Society*, trans by John Wilkinson, New York, Alfred A Knopf, 1964. In my discussion of computers and power here I am particularly indebted to Langdon Winner, *The Whale and the Reactor. A Search for Limits in an Age of High Technology.* Chicago/London, Chicago University Press, 1986, and to Stephen L Talbott, *The Future Does Not Compute. Transcending The Machines in Our Midst.* Sebastopol, Calif, O'Reilly & Associates, 1995. See also, Ivan Illich, *Limits to Medicine: Medical Nemesis, The Expropriation of Health*, London, Marion Boyars, 1995 (enlarged edition). On dilemmas discussed here see also John Gray, *After Social Democracy*, London, Demos, Paper No. 18, 1996. For the research background to what patients say see the King's Fund Development Centre's *Promoting Patient Choice* project. Also, contributions to *But Will It Work, Doctor? 1996* conference, King's Fund/NHS Executive &c, Northampton, 22 May 1996 (in press), especially Angela Coulter, "Developing evidence-based patient choice"; Mary Newburn, "Challenging the traditional doctor/patient relationship", Sandy Oliver, "Involving consumers in generating evidence", and Lesley Fallowfield, "Making decisions about treatments: how do patients with cancer choose?", and my keynote address: "But will it work *for me*, doctor?" See also Ann Cull, "What do quality of life measures show", address to *Cancer Services: From Calman to the Millennium*, conference, NHS Executive West Midlands, Birmingham, 9 May 1996, and *"Patient-Centred Cancer Services? What Patients Say*, Oxford, National Cancer Alliance, May 1996. Also, Leeds, *NHS Magazine*, 5, Summer, 1996, Lynne Greenwood and Lynn May, "A question of choice".

2 Marshall Marinker, "The End of General Practice", The 1994 Bayliss Lecture, London, November 1994; Bruce Mazlish, *The Fourth Discontinuity. The Co-Evolution of Humans and Machines.* New Haven and London, Yale University Press, 1993, p 14.

3 Tony Hope, "Doctors and Patients Talking", address to *But Will It Work, Doctor? 1996* conference, King's Fund/NHS Executive &c, Northampton, 22 May 1996. It will be useful to assess the arguments of this interesting paper once the audit of professional behaviour is known from the use made of the *Informed Choice* initiative (launched on 18 January 1996 by the NHS Centre for Reviews and Dissemination and the Midwives Information and Resource Service). The results of the innovative King's Fund Development Centre's *Promoting Patient Choice* project, promoting both concepts and materials for patient choice, already show that patient's capacity for choice has been under-estimated, and that very significant gains can result. For the NHS, however, "information" and "choice" are not the same thing, and there is no consistency in either. Geography, race, gender, age, mental health state, physical mobility, class and education all intrude, as well as professional attitude and basic systems deficits. See Lynne Greenwood and Lynn May report, op cit.

4 Marshall Marinker, "Beyond Management", speech to Institute of Health Services Management annual conference, Harrogate, June 1995.

5 AJ Cullyer, "Chisels or Screwdrivers? A Critique of the NERA proposals for the reform of the NHS", in A Towse (ed), *Financing Health Care in the UK*, London, Office of Health Economics, 1995.

6 David B Friend, "Real world health care needs", Boston, Mass, *Watson Wyatt Communicator*, Fall/Winter 1995; "Health Care in the Year 2020", *Watson Wyatt Insights*, Boston, Mass, Winter 1995; Innovation Centre for Information Technology in the Enterprise, Unit of Harvard Medical School and Brigham & Women's Hospital, Boston, MA. Decision Systems Group brochure, 1996.

7 Marilyn M Rosenthal, *The Incompetent Doctor, Behind Closed Doors*. Buckingham Open University Press, 1995; Tavs Folmer Andersen and Gavin Mooney (eds), *The Challenges of Medical Practice Variations*, London, Macmillan Press, 1990.

8 David Green argues that one means for the consumer to adapt to uncertainty and the lack of information is to employ Doctors directly, as they did in Friendly Societies until the changes in 1911 and in 1948. See David G Green, *Working Class Patients and the Medical Establishment*, London, Temple Smith, 1985. See also his argument that patients are not "an interest" within the NHS, but the reason for its existence, in "Note of Dissent", Minority Report, in *UK Healthcare Services, Challenges and Policy Options, A Report by Healthcare 2000*, 19 September 1995.

9 See Introduction to my *The Invisible Hospital and the Secret Garden, An Insider's Commentary on the NHS Reforms* (Abingdon, Radcliffe Medical Press/Institute of Health Services Management, 1995).

10 "Keeping Going", in Seamus Heaney, *The Spirit Level*, London, Faber & Faber, 1996.

11 JM Synge, *The Playboy of the Western World* (1907); See my *The Invisible Hospital and the Secret Garden*, op cit. Also, Christopher M Ward, "Rights and Wrongs of Being a Surgeon", *Surgery*, 1995, pp 176–8, and Ian Kendall and Graham Moon, "Health Policy and the Conservatives", in Stephen P Savage, Rob Atkinson, and Lynton Robins (eds) *Public Policy in Britain*, London, Macmillan, 1994. Also, London, Department of Health, *Patient Partnership: Building a Collaborative Strategy*, July 1996; Department of Health, *Priorities and Planning Guidance for the NHS: 1997/98*, London, Department of Health, June 1996. I hope to offer an extended discussion of these issues in my *"The Prison of Awe": Patients and Power* (in preparation).

12 Private conversation with Perri 6, London, June 1996. This work is forthcoming in the Demos *Arguments* series.

13 I owe this revelatory phrase to John Simmonds; private conversation, July 1996.

14 Isaiah Berlin, *Four Essays on Liberty*, Oxford, Oxford University Press, 1969; Ramin Jahanbegloo, *Conversations with Isaiah Berlin. Recollections of an Historian of Ideas*, London, Peter Halban, 1992; John Gray, *Berlin*, London, Fontana Press, 1995. Also, the invaluable commentary by David G Green, "Note of Dissent", Minority Report, in *UK Healthcare Services, Challenges and Policy Options, A Report by Healthcare 2000*, op cit; FA Hayek, *The Fatal Conceit*, London, Routledge, 1988. Also, my *Who Owns Our Bodies?* (Abingdon, Radcliffe Medical Press/Institute for Health Policy Studies, 1996).

15 Healthcare in the year 2020 *Watson Wyatt Insights* 1995, Winter.

16 Sue Roe, "Shelving the Self", in S Roe, Susan Sellars, Nicole Warde Jouve, and Michele Roberts, *The Semi-Transparent Envelope. Women Writing—Feminism and Fiction*, London/New York, Marion Boyars, 1994, p 65.

17 Alvin Toffler, *Future Shock*, London, The Bodley Head, 1970, p 11.

18 Philip Kitcher, *The Lives to Come. The Genetic Revolution and Human Possibilities.* London, Allen Lane/The Penguin Press, 1996.

19 David G Green, *Community Without Politics, A Market Approach to Welfare Reform*, London, IEA Health and Welfare Unit, 1996. See also, on local democracy, Gray, op cit.

20 Winner, op cit, p 93.

21 Winner, ibid, p 55.

22 Mazlish, op cit, p 8.

23 Quoted in Mazlish, ibid, p 87.

24 See the introduction to my *The Invisible Hospital and the Secret Garden* for a further discussion. For public choice theory, or the economics of politics of the "Virginia School of Public Choice", see James Buchanan and Gordon Tullock, *The Calculus of Consent*, Ann Arbor, Michigan, University of Michigan Press, 1965; J Buchanan (ed) *The Economics of Politics*, London, Institute of Economic Affairs, 1978; James Buchanan, *The Limits of Liberty: Between Anarchy and*

Leviathan, Chicago, University of Chicago Press, 1975; Gordon Tullock, *The Vote Motive*, London, IEA, 1976; Arthur Seldon, *Capitalism*, Oxford, Basil Blackwell, 1990, and Peter Self, *Government by the Market? The Politics of Public Choice*, London, Macmillan, 1993.

25 Harold Inniss, quoted in Tapscott, op cit, p 386.

26 Nicholas Negroponte, *Being Digital*, London, Hodder & Stoughton, 1995; Don Tapscott, *The Digital Economy. Promise and Peril in the Age of Networked Intelligence*, New York, McGraw Hill, 1996; Bill Gates (with Nathan Myhrvold and Peter Rinearson), *The Road Ahead*, London, Viking, 1995; Roy Lilley, *Futureproofing*, Abingdon, The Radcliffe Press, 1995. Also, Mazlish, ibid. For specific applications in medicine, see *Proceedings of Telemed 95, Medicine on the Superhighway. International Conference on Telemedicine and Telecare*, London, 8–9 November 1995, *Journal of Telemedicine and Telecare*, 2, Supplement 1, 1996.

27 Iona Heath, *The Mystery of Medical Practice*, London, Nuffield Provincial Hospitals Trust, 1995, p 3.

28 Heath, ibid, p 3.

29 Jane Austen, *Northanger Abbey*, London, 1818, Chapter V.

30 Heath, op cit.

31 Thomas McKeown, *The Role of Medicine: Dream, Mirage or Nemesis*, Oxford, Basil Blackwell, 1979; Robert G Evans, Morris L Barer, and Theodore R Marmor, *Why Are Some People Healthy and Others Not?* New York, Aldine de Gruyter, 1994; Robert G Evans, "The dog in the night-time: Medical practice variations and health policy", in Tavs Folmer Andersen and Gavin Mooney (eds), *The Challenges of Medical Practice Variations*, op cit; Leonard A Sagan, *The Health of Nations*, New York, Basic Books, 1987; John B McKinlay and Sonja M McKinlay, "The Questionable Contribution of Medical Measures to the Decline of Mortality in the United States in the Twentieth Century", *Milbank Memorial Fund Quarterly*, Health and Society, 55, 3, Summer 1977. Also, Edward Tenner, *Why Things Bite Back. Technology and the Revenge Effect*, London, Fourth Estate, 1996 for a valuable discussion and a provocative context.

32 Peter M Senge, *The Fifth Discipline. The Art and Practice of the Learning Organisation.* New York, Doubleday, 1990.

33 Negroponte, op cit, p 47.

34 Langdon Winner, *The Whale and the Reactor. A Search for Limits in an Age of High Technology.* Chicago/London, Chicago University Press, 1986, p ix.

35 Peter F Drucker, "The Age of Social Transformation", *Atlantic Monthly*, November 1994.

36 David G Green, *Community Without Politics, A Market Approach to Welfare Reform*, London, IEA Health and Welfare Unit, 1996 and *Reinventing Civil Society*, London, IEA, 1993.

37 Lewis Mumford, *The Myth of the Machine: The Pentagon of Power*, New York, Harcourt Brace Jovanovich, 1970; Herbert Marcuse, *One-Dimensional Man: Studies in the Ideology of Advanced Industrial Society*, Boston, Beacon Press, 1964; Jacques Ellul, *The Technological Society*, trans by John Wilkinson, New York, Alfred A Knopf, 1964; Jerry Mander, *In the Absence of the Sacred. The Failure of Technology and The Survival of the Indian Nations*, San Francisco, Sierra Club Books, 1991; Theodore Roszak, *The Making of a Counter Culture; Reflections on Technocratic Society and its Youthful Opposition*, Garden City, New York, Doubleday, 1969; Theodore Roszak, *The Cult of Information. A Neo-Luddite Treatise on High-Tech, Artificial Intelligence, and The Art of True Thinking*, Berkeley, University of California Press, second edition, 1994; Stephen L Talbott, *The Future Does Not Compute. Transcending The Machines in Our Midst.* Sebastopol, Calif, O'Reilly & Associates, 1995, Anthony Smith, *Software for the self. Culture*

and Technology, TS Eliot Lectures, 1994. London, Faber and Faber, 1995; Clifford Stoll, *Silicon Snake Oil. Second Thoughts on the Information Highway,* London, Macmillan, 1995; also, Mazlish, ibid, and Winner, ibid.

38 Winner, op cit, p 9.

39 Winner, ibid, p 17.

40 Cited in Paul Theroux, *The Great Railway Bazaar,* op cit, p [6].

41 See the extraordinarily prescient article by Marshall Marinker, "The Future of Medicine: 2010", London, *Journal of the Royal College of General Practitioners,* 1981, 31, pp 540–546. Also, Edmund Faltermayer, "Health Care: Building the System We Need", New York, *Fortune Magazine,* 23 March 1992, and Alexandria Wyke, "The Future of Medicine", Peering Into 2010, London, *The Economist,* 19 March 1994. Also, addresses to Royal College of Physicians conference, London, 12 July 1996: Uwe Reinhardt, "The changing economics of health care"; James Halls, "Telemedicine and teleradiology—the University of Southern California experience"; C Forbes Dewey Jr, "Information technology in health care"; Mark Ferguson, "The UK Technology Foresight Programme".

42 *The Financial Times,* London, *FT Review of Information Technology,* February 1996, for sources of product data, innovation and discussion of technical developments, amongst many other current-affairs sources crowded with "On-Line" news. Also, Bruce C McKenzie, *Medicine and the Internet. Introducing Online Resources and Terminology.* Oxford, Oxford University Press, 1996.

43 Winner, op cit, p 56.

44 London, Department of Health, NHS Executive, Information Management Group publications: *A Strategy for NHS-wide networking,* August 1994; *NHS-wide networking programme, Security guide for IM&T specialists,* November 1995; *Implementing the infrastructure, A Handbook for IM&T specialists,* March 1996; *Programmes and Projects Information Pack,* June 1996; also, Department of Health, EL (95) 108: *Security in the NHS-Wide Networking System,* 6 December 1995; FHS Computer Unit, *Annual Report and Accounts, 1994–95,* Exeter, December 1995. On security concerns, see London, Department of Health, *The Protection and Use of Patient Information, Guidance from the Department of Health,* 7 March 1996; also, Ross J Anderson, *Security in Clinical Information Systems,* London, BMA, January 1996; Ross Anderson, "Clinical system security: interim guidelines", London, *British Medical Journal,* 312, 13 January 1996, pp 109–11.

45 Andrea J Smith and Catherine A Godfrey, *IRIS, An Interactive Computer System for Monitoring and Improving Quality from the Patient's Perspective,* Camden & Islington Community Health Services NHS Trust, May 1996; "Update on the Virtual World", London, *Research in Action,* Summer 1996, p 11.

46 Perri 6 and Ivan Briscoe, *On the Cards. Privacy, identity and trust in the age of Smart Card Technologies.* London, Demos, Paper No 20, 1996; Geoff Mulgan and Ivan Briscoe, *The Society of Networks: A New Model for the Information Superhighway and the communications supermarket.* London, Demos, Arguments Series, 5, 1995; *The Information Society: Getting it Right for Consumers,* London, National Consumer Council, 1996.

47 Jean Miles, "Computer solace", London, *The Financial Times,* 25/26 May 1996; Sally Neale, "Surfer, heal thyself", London, *The Guardian,* 20 September 1995. See also, Margaret JA Edwards, *The Internet, For Nurses and Allied Health Professionals,* New York, Springer, 1995.

48 JF Kasper, AG Mulley and JE Wennberg, "Developing Shared Decision-Making Programs to Improve the Quality of Health Care," *Quality Review Bulletin,* Vol 18, No 6, 1992, pp 182–90; also, Adam Darkins, "Shared Decision Making in Health Care Systems", in *Proceedings from the Annual Research Conference 1994, Profession business or trade: do the professions have a future?* The Law Society Research and Planning Unit, London, 1994.

49 *The Information Society*, op cit.
50 Rudolf Klein, *The New Politics of the National Health Service*, London, Longman, Third edition, 1995.
51 *Health Service Commissioner Annual Report for 1994/95*, London, HMSO, 1995 (July); *Health Service Commissioner Annual Report for 1995/96*, London, HMSO, 1996 (June); Audit Commission, *What Seems To Be The Matter: Communication Between Hospitals and Patients*, London, HMSO, 1993. See also J Bradburn &c, "Eye Opener", *The Health Service Journal*. August 4 1994, pp 20–21. Compare American consumer data and approaches. For example, the guide to Washington, DC area hospitals, *Washington Consumer's Checkbook*; Gambone JC, Reiter RC, *Prepared for Health Care, A Consumer's Guide to Medical Decisions*, Great Performance Inc, Beavertton, Oregon, 1993. On hospital quality assessment, patient outcomes and patient satisfaction measures for 29 hospitals in Cleveland, Ohio, see *Cleveland Health Quality Choice Summary Report*, April 1993–half-yearly since; Gary E Rosenthal and Dwain L Harper, "Cleveland Health Quality Choice: A Model for Collaborative Community-Based Outcomes assessment", *Joint Commission Journal of Quality Improvement*, 20, 8, 1994; and Gary E Rosenthal, Linda Quinn and Dwain L Harper, "Declines in Hospital Mortality Associated with a Regional Initiative to Measure Hospital Performance" (in press).
52 Marinker, IHSM, op cit.
53 Marshall Marinker, "The End of General Practice", op cit. See also, Diane Plamping, "A Service Development Perspective", address to primary care conference, Making it Happen: Learning from local solutions, King's Fund, Gateshead, 21 May 1996. On suitability of GPs and primary care-led NHS see Steve Iliffe, "The retreat from equity: implications of the shift towards a primary-care led NHS", *Critical Public Health*, 1995, 6, 3, pp 36–42. Also, Heath, op cit.
54 Tenner, op cit, p 21.
55 Tenner, ibid, p 26.
56 Tenner, ibid, p 51.
57 Tenner, ibid, p 277.
58 Harry Burns, *Making Outcomes Matter*, Birmingham, NAHAT, 'Speaking Up' series, no 5, January 1996. Based on speech to NAHAT Annual Conference, Glasgow, June 1995.
59 See SH Heap &c, *The Theory of Choice*, Oxford, Blackwell, 1992. Also, Samuel Brittan, "Some ruminations on risk", London, *The Financial Times*, 11 April 1996, p 12.
60 Shoshana Zuboff, *In the Age of the Smart Machine*, New York, Basic Books, 1988.
61 Tapscott, op cit, p 75.
62 Tapscott, ibid, p 87.
63 Tapscott, op cit, p 188.
64 Tapscott, ibid, p 27.
65 Karen Pallario, "Virtual Healthcare, New York, *Modern Healthcare*, 18 March 1996.
66 Perri 6 and Ivan Briscoe, op cit, p 6. Also, Geoff Mulgan and I Briscoe, op cit.
67 G Mulgan and I Briscoe, ibid.
68 Paul Hodgkin, "Information technology, rapid change and the NHS". Draft Paper for the Framework for Appropriate Care Throughout Sheffield Project, May 1995, p 5.
69 Neil Belton, "Candied Porkers: British Scorn of the Scientific", in Francis Spufford and Jenny Uglow (eds) *Cultural Babbage. Technology, Time and Invention*. London, Faber and Faber, 1996, p 240.

70 See Rose Echlin with Judith Buck, *Partners in Change. Care Planning in Mental Health Services*, London, King's Fund, 1995.

71 Jenny Uglow, "Introduction: 'Possibility' ", in Francis Spufford and Jenny Uglow, op cit.

72 WE Gladstone, *Studies on Homer*, quoted in Jasper Griffin, *Homer*, Oxford, Oxford University Press, 1996, p 1; Charles Darwin, *The Origin of Species*, London, John Murray, 1859.

73 James Joyce, *Ulysses*, London, Penguin edition, introduction by Declan Kiberd, 1992, p. 38.

74 Perri 6, "Governing by cultures", London, *Demos Quarterly*, 7, 1995, pp. 2–8.

75 Joyce, *Ulysses*, p. 30. See also, on what is possible, a series of important, short articles which offer a subtle commentary on "beneficial patient care", and on patient responsibility/satisfaction: William G. Pickering: " 'Patient care' and patient benefit" (letter), *J. of the Royal College of General Practitioners*, September 1989, p. 389; "A nation of people called patients", *J. of Medical Ethics*, 1991, 17, pp. 91–2; "Patient satisfaction: an imperfect measurement of quality medicine", *J. of Medical Ethics*, 1993, pp. 121–2; "Kindness, prescribed and natural in medical practice" (in press). Also, for a critique of what the NHS measures and does not measure (or seek to secure by contract), John Flemming and Peter Oppenheimer, "Are Government Spending and Taxes Too High (or Too Low)?, London, *National Institute Economic Review*, 157, July 1996, pp. 57–76. On NHS "progress" on the Internet, and the conspicuous absence of quality data offered by Trusts on the Net, see Dan Jellinek, "Slow Start on the Super-highway", *Healthcare Today*, September 1996, pp. 24–5 and "Net progress", p. 22.

76 Jane Austen, *Mansfield Park*, 1814, Chapter 1; *Northanger Abbey*, Chapter 1.

77 William Shakespeare, *Troilus and Cressida*, Act 3, Scene 2.

Index